FACE YOGA

SCULPT, LIFT & TONE IN JUST 10 MINUTES A DAY

ANASTASIA GORON

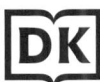

Introduction 04
How I Got Here 06

Understand Your Face 08

The Hidden Architecture 10
Your Face Map 34
Self-Analyse Your Face 36

The Method & Movements 40

The All You Can Face Method 42
How to Build Your Routine 44
Before You Begin 46

Phase 01
Posture Practice 48

Phase 02
Release Tension 74

Phase 03
Strengthen 120

The Routines 162

Combat Tired Eyes 164
Combat Puffy Eyes 166
Combat Drooping Eyelids 168
Combat Frown Lines 170

Combat Sagging Cheeks 172
Combat Smile Lines 174
Combat Thinning Lips 176
Combat a Drooping Mouth 178
Combat Jaw Tension 180
Combat a Double Chin 182
Combat a Sagging Neck 184
Combat Facial Asymmetry 186
Combat Dull Skin 188
Combat Tension Headache 190
Combat Puffiness 192

The Tools 194

Supporting Tools 196
Gua Sha 197
Facial Cups 198
Acupuncture Pen 199
Spoons 200
Jade Roller 201

Conclusion 202
Recommended Reading 203
Index 204
References 206
Acknowledgements 207
About the Author 208

Introduction
Dear Reader

Pause for a moment. Look at yourself in the mirror. Truly look. What is the first thought that crosses your mind? Is it kind? Is it curious? Or is it quietly critical, shaped by years of subtle messages telling you how you should look, rather than inviting you to see how magnificent you already are?

For most of us, that inner voice is far harsher than we deserve. We live in a world that constantly tells us we aren't enough. That we should chase youth. That we should fix, hide, or improve ourselves to belong. The beauty industry thrives on this – selling endless solutions for imagined flaws, offering promises of perfection through creams, procedures, filters, and edits. And all the while, the quiet pressure grows to change yourself so you can be worthy.

But what if the opposite is true? What if the face you see in the mirror is not a problem to solve, but a map to read? What if the so-called flaws that worry you – lines, puffiness, and asymmetries – are not defects at all, but symptoms? What if they're clues from your body, signalling how you hold tension, how you move, how you breathe, how you feel? And what if, by learning to listen to these clues, you could rejuvenate your face, reduce wrinkles, eliminate puffiness, improve facial asymmetry, and gain your confidence back, not by fighting against yourself, but by working *with* your body's natural design?

Your face is your first language

It speaks to the world in micro-movements, expressions, and subtle shifts. Science shows that up to ninety-three per cent of communication is non-verbal.[1] Every lift of your brow, softening of your eyes, or pull of your lips sends signals about who you are and how you feel.

And yet, modern culture encourages us to erase these signals. To freeze, paralyze, or smooth them in the name of "beauty". But studies in social neuroscience reveal that facial expressiveness is central to human connection. When we block it, we dampen empathy, trust, and emotional resonance.[2]

In a time when loneliness and disconnection are rising at alarming rates – with the World Health Organization[3] naming loneliness a major public health concern, losing this form of communication – which is profoundly human – is more than aesthetic.

What you see in the mirror is not random

Every line, fold, or hollow you see in your face is the result of deeper forces. A forward head posture for example, which is common from screen use, can double or triple the load on your neck and jaw,[4] pulling your face downwards, deepening folds, and creating puffiness. Similarly, tight fascia and muscle patterns lock in tension (which you'll learn more about in Part One), which etches itself into the skin over time,[5] causing creases to deepen, features to shift, and the face to lose its natural mobility and glow.

What we're taught to think of as flaws are often visible symptoms caused by deeper imbalances in structure, tension, and flow. And here lies your power: when you address those root causes, you don't just change how your face looks – you change how you feel.

This book is not about "anti-aging"

The very idea of anti-aging is, in truth, absurd. Aging is a privilege. Every year, every change in your face tells the story of who you are and what you've lived. This book will not offer you ways to deny that. Instead, it will offer ways to become the most vibrant, alive, and authentic version of yourself at any age.

My method is not about looking like someone else. It's about seeing your face – and yourself – clearly, and about moving from critique to care. It's about achieving the real, visible results that matter: rejuvenating your face, softening lines, eliminating puffiness, improving symmetry, and regaining confidence through daily rituals that respect your body.

Face yoga, as you'll practise it here, is not just about changing your reflection. It's about changing your relationship with your reflection, and about making peace with the face that has carried you through joy, struggle, and growth.

Every exercise, every technique, is an invitation to listen more deeply. To soften the harsh inner voice.

A personal invitation

When I began this journey, like many, I believed face yoga was about looking younger. But the daily practice of touch, breath, and attention changed not just my face, but my heart. The more I connected with myself, the kinder my inner voice became. And the more my face reflected this inner change – looking brighter, smoother, more alive – the more my confidence grew.

And that is my hope for you: that this book inspires you to take action, not out of fear, but out of love. That it gives you clarity, not confusion. That it helps you build not just a more vibrant face, but a more compassionate relationship with yourself – and with the world around you.

With love,
Anastasia Goron
Founder, All You Can Face

How I Got Here

A Challenging Start

I was born in Ukraine and spent my early childhood in Germany, growing up in a refugee camp. We shared a bathroom with eight other families. Safety, stability, privacy – these weren't things I could count on. But my parents did everything they could to shield me. They believed that education, discipline, and culture could help me rise above our circumstances.

At five, I was enrolled in one of Europe's most prestigious ballet schools – a place that prepared girls to become prima ballerinas. From the start, my body was measured, judged, compared. I learned resilience. But I also learned to ask myself, quietly but persistently: *Am I enough?*

I danced intensely until I was fifteen – always the tallest, often feeling like the awkward one beside my peers. When an agent suggested I try modelling, I thought it was just because of my height. I didn't see myself as beautiful. But I stepped into that world – hoping, perhaps, to finally feel like I belonged.

Instead, the scrutiny deepened. My forehead was too big. My nose too prominent. My calves too muscular. My skin too pale – or not pale enough. I learned to smile through it, to fake confidence, to wear a mask. But inside, I absorbed every word until their critiques became my inner voice.

Modelling let me travel the world, meet inspiring creatives, see cities I never imagined visiting. But no matter how much I achieved, I felt like an imposter – as if my worth was fragile, conditional, always on trial. And my acne only compounded the struggle. I tried every promise the beauty industry sold – but nothing brought peace with my reflection.

Everything changed the day my mother invited me to a face yoga class. I had no idea what it was. I went because I had nothing else to do that weekend. I was the youngest person there by decades. But the teacher's face – radiant, balanced, glowing – caught my attention.

As I followed the exercises, I felt something I hadn't felt in years: connection. I looked better, yes – but I also felt better. I felt like I'd uncovered a secret that no one was talking about.

From that day on, I became obsessed. I spent years learning in every free moment. I read surgical anatomy books and researched fascia. I studied orthodontics, dermatology, Traditional Chinese Medicine, and myofascial release. I sought out experts – especially in cultures where facial exercises and massage weren't trends, but tradition.

I practised, observed, refined. I experimented. I wasn't learning to chase perfection – I was learning to reconnect with myself. And slowly, I felt the harsh voice in my head begin to soften.

One day, a friend and I filmed a funny birthday video for someone we loved. I wasn't thinking about how I looked. If anything, I felt self-conscious.

But afterwards, my friend called and asked, "What did you do to your face? You look amazing."

He didn't give compliments lightly. He didn't believe me at first when I said: "It's face yoga."

That's when I knew: it wasn't just me who felt the change – others saw it too.

In 2020, I finally began sharing it, creating my brand and method, All You Can Face. I had no business plan – just a desire to see if others felt drawn to this practice as I did.

The response was overwhelming. People from around the world connected – not just with the idea of changing how they looked, but of reconnecting with themselves. They said things such as:

"I wear my hair back now. I used to hide my face."

"I'm 40, going through chemo, and people think I'm 26. It's the face yoga."

"My husband keeps asking what I'm doing. I look younger every day."

That's when I realized: this was bigger than me.

I'm not here to tell you Botox or surgery is wrong. I believe in choice. But too many people don't even know face yoga is an option. My hope is that this book opens that door for you.

Face yoga isn't magic. It's not a quick fix. It's a method. A practice. A way to build trust with yourself and feel at home in your skin.

And if it helped me, I believe it can help you too. In these pages, I'll show you how.

My method grew from wanting change, and the discovery that knowledge and compassion helps us transform our faces with our own hands.

UNDERSTAND

YOUR FACE

The Hidden Architecture

The Anatomy of Your Face

Your face is more than just what you see in the mirror – it's a complex, functional system made up of many interconnected parts. Glowing skin, puffy features, or folds are the result of an intricate dance happening beneath the surface. To truly understand how facial training works – and why it works – you need to understand what's beneath the surface.

Face yoga targets seven key components of the face: skin, fat, muscles, fascia, nerves, blood and lymph, and bone. These are the building blocks of expression, tone, and glow.

These parts never work in isolation. They are deeply interconnected, which is why one pull, blockage, or habit can affect your entire appearance. This is why your face can't be "fixed" from the outside in – it needs a systematic approach.

Once you understand how your face actually works, you can begin to work with it, not against it. You don't need machines, needles, or expensive creams. Just awareness, consistency, and the power of your hands.

Skin
The Reflective Surface

Your skin is your face's most visible layer, but it's also the most misunderstood. It's your largest organ, and it communicates with you daily. Often treated as the starting point for beauty and time-related changes, your skin is actually the *result* of what's happening underneath. Facial skin is thinner, more expressive, and more sensitive than skin on most other parts of the body. It reflects your inner health, hydration, circulation, and muscle tone, and is a powerful messenger. Instead of masking symptoms, you can learn to listen to them.

Fat
The Volume and Contour Shaper

Fat is not your enemy. In fact, fat is youth. Facial fat isn't just about "fullness"; it plays a vital role in shaping and supporting your face. Beneath the skin, fat pads are arranged in defined compartments, either above or between muscles. These compartments help create the smooth curves of your cheeks, the under-eye area, and the fullness around your temples and jawline.

Muscles
The Movers of Emotion and Form

Your face contains more than 40 muscles (see page 18), many of which are mimetic, meaning they connect directly to the skin on one end and anchor to bone on the other. This anatomical setup allows the muscle to pull the skin when the muscle contracts. This unique structure – where the muscle anchors to bone on one end and attaches to the skin on the other – gives rise to every subtle movement, creating visible changes. This connection explains how micro-expressions emerge: a twitch of the eyebrow, a subtle smile, a lifted cheek.

Fascia
The Web That Connects Everything

Fascia is the most underestimated tissue in the body, and yet, it might be the most important when it comes to understanding facial structure and function. It's a thin, elastic web of connective tissue that wraps around every muscle, nerve, organ, and bone. Thomas Myers, author of *Anatomy Trains*,[1] describes fascia as part of a continuous, body-wide network of myofascial lines (continuous bands of connective tissue that are like stretchy, interconnected threads of fabric that weave through your entire body) that run from head to toe.

Nerves
The Face's Emotional Highway

Your face is one of the most neurologically dense areas in the body. It's wired directly to the brainstem via the cranial nerves, especially the facial nerve (CN VII), which controls most expression muscles, and the trigeminal nerve (CN V), which handles sensation in the face. Facial expressions are not just conscious – they're reflexive. Stress, trauma, or emotional memories can create long-standing patterns in facial tone and posture.[6] But the connection also flows in reverse. Just as emotions shape our expressions, consciously softening the face can influence the nervous system – a concept often used in somatic therapies.

Blood and Lymph
The Face's Flow System

Every cell in your face depends on one thing: flow. Your circulatory system (the network of organs and blood vessels that circulate blood throughout your body) brings fresh oxygen and nutrients, while your lymphatic system (the group of organs, vessels, and tissues that protect you from infection, and keep a balance of fluids flowing throughout your body) removes waste and toxins. Together, they are the lifelines of your skin, muscles, and overall facial health.

Bone
The Silent Sculptor

Underneath every expression and movement there is structure: bone. Many facial muscles originate or anchor on bones, so their function depends on stable bone structure. And it goes both ways – just as bone influences muscle tone and alignment, consistent muscular activity also stimulates bone remodelling through mechanical tension. When muscle tone is balanced and functional, it helps maintain healthy pressure on the bone, encouraging strength and density through natural movement. Bone may be the deepest layer, but it's far from passive. Aid your bone structure from the outside – with movement, flow, and balance – and it will support the rest of your face from within.

What Your Face Is Trying to Tell You

We've been taught to fear the signs of aging. A wrinkle is something to erase. A sagging jawline is something to lift. And puffy eyes? There's a solution for that. But what if these so-called flaws were never the real issue? What if they were simply the surface expressions of deeper imbalances – whispers from your body, asking to be heard?

The beauty industry has conditioned us to respond to every change in our face with a surface fix. But these fixes rarely last, because they don't reach the root. They're like painting over a crack in the wall without fixing the foundation. You might feel better momentarily, but the underlying problem is still there, waiting to be heard. And unless we pause to ask *why* these changes are happening in the first place, we'll stay stuck in the loop of chasing symptoms.

CHANGE IN THE FACE	WHAT WE USUALLY DO
Loss of facial contours and double chin	Apply lifting creams, use facial tape, or undergo laser tightening treatments
Puffy eyes and morning facial swelling	Use cold tools or eye serums
Dull or tired-looking skin	Apply brightening serums or strong exfoliants
Deep expression lines	Fill or freeze lines with injectables or apply anti-aging creams
Mid-face hollowing and drooping cheeks	Use fillers or contouring makeup
Facial asymmetry or uneven texture	Try microneedling, lasers, or surgery
Flattened or collapsing cheeks	Use contouring products or blush
Pronounced nasolabial folds	Use filler to lift or mask the fold
Hooded or drooping eyelids	Apply firming eye creams or consider blepharoplasty

WHAT THE ACTUAL CAUSE IS	WHY IT DOESN'T HELP
Poor posture, tight fascia, low tongue position, and bone remodelling	Doesn't address posture, fascia, or muscular support causing descent
Blocked lymphatic drainage due to poor posture and fascial congestion	Doesn't activate lymph flow or fix blocked drainage pathways
Sluggish blood flow, chronic stress, and impaired nutrient delivery	Only addresses the surface; it doesn't improve circulation or stress
Chronic muscle tension and emotional expression patterns	Ignores the muscle patterns and emotional tension causing the lines
Loss of internal support from posture, tongue position, fat pad descent, and bone density decline	Treats the symptom, not the weak posture or internal support loss
Muscle imbalance, dominant movement patterns, and fascial asymmetry	Doesn't resolve underlying tension, dominance, or compensation
Bone resorption, muscle disuse, and fascial dryness	Only masks visual loss of lift from bone loss and muscle disuse
Descent of cheek fat pads, weakened zygomatic muscles, facial tension pulling downwards, and chronic masseter tension, which causes skin to fold	Filler may add volume short term but doesn't address the sagging caused by structural collapse and muscle imbalance
Overworked frontalis muscle, chronic neck tension, brow tension, and loss of support from forehead and scalp fascia	Topical treatments don't affect muscular tension or fascial restrictions that are pulling the eyelid area down

Postural Imbalances

The Anatomy Behind Posture & Facial Aging

Your head weighs around 5 kilograms (11 pounds). Imagine balancing a bowling ball on top of your spine all day! In perfect alignment, your bones, muscles, and joints carry this effortlessly. But tilt your head forwards just 2-3 centimetres (1 inch), and that weight doubles or even triples in strain. This common condition is known as "forward head posture", or "tech neck".

When Posture Collapses

1. **Blood flow gets compromised**
   A forward head and rounded shoulders compresses the arteries in the neck that deliver oxygen and nutrients to your skin.
   Result *dull skin, slower cell turnover, early signs of aging*

2. **Lymphatic drainage slows down**
   Poor posture compresses critical drainage zones.
   Result *puffiness around the eyes, jawline, and cheeks*

3. **Fascia and muscle imbalances lock in aging**
   Postural shifts change how fascia distributes tension. Over time, your body adapts, reinforcing slouching and creating downwards pull on your face.
   Result *marionette lines, nasolabial folds, jowls*

THE POSTURE-FACE CONNECTION IN ACTION

Posture	Symptoms
Tech neck	Double chin and jawline blur
Rounded shoulders	Puffy face and poor lymph flow
Collapsed chest	Dull skin tone and fatigued look
Forward head	Deepened nasolabial folds and jowls

Key Players in Postural Anatomy

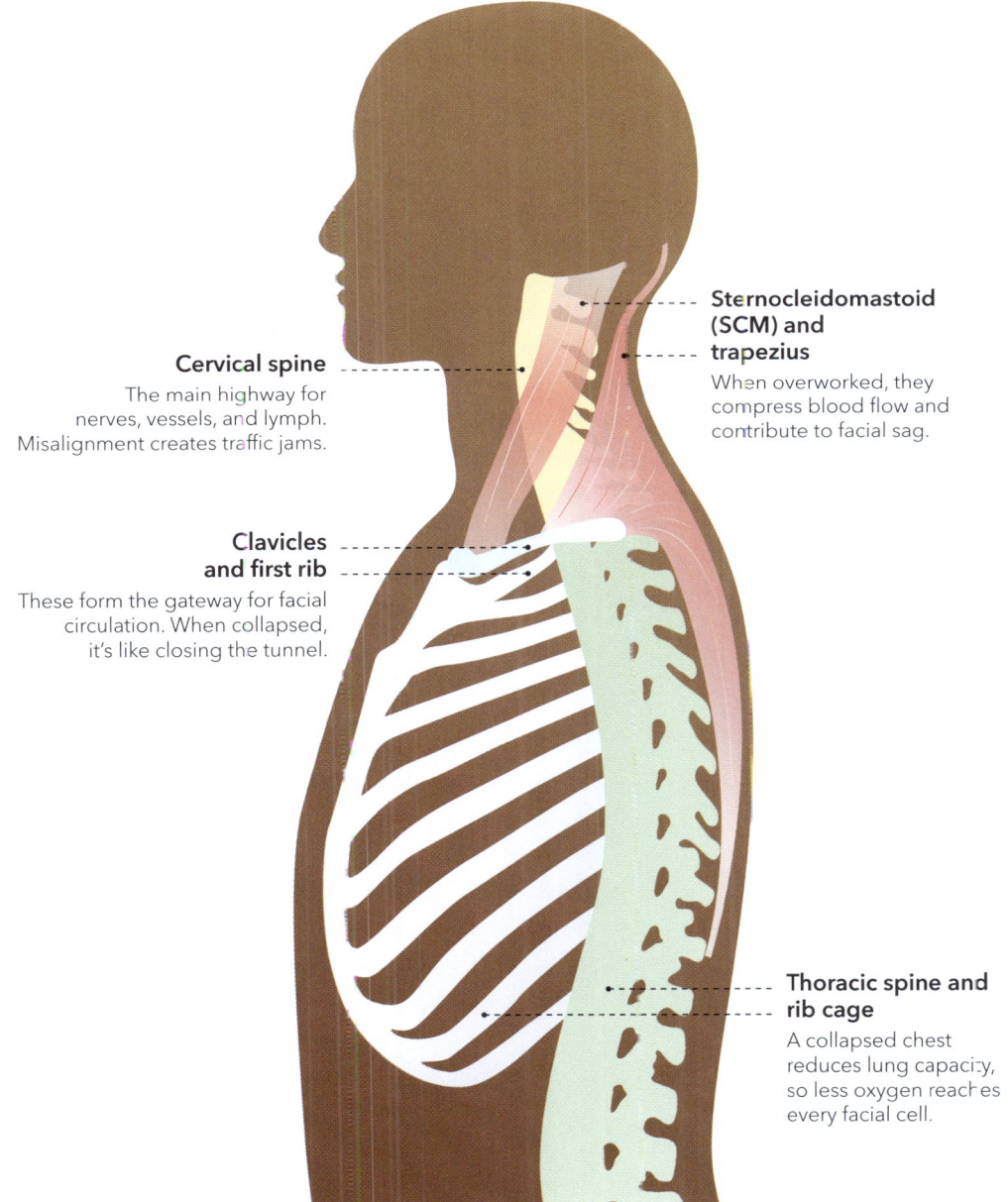

Cervical spine
The main highway for nerves, vessels, and lymph. Misalignment creates traffic jams.

Sternocleidomastoid (SCM) and trapezius
When overworked, they compress blood flow and contribute to facial sag.

Clavicles and first rib
These form the gateway for facial circulation. When collapsed, it's like closing the tunnel.

Thoracic spine and rib cage
A collapsed chest reduces lung capacity, so less oxygen reaches every facial cell.

Fascia & Muscle Tension

The Anatomy Behind Tension & Your Face

Fascia is the connective tissue web that helps keep everything in place. But when you're stressed, still, dehydrated, or holding repeated tension, it stiffens and loses its glide, which starts pulling on your features like strings on a marionette.

Imagine pulling on the hem of a bedsheet. Wrinkles and stress points appear across the entire surface. Your fascia behaves similarly. If your neck or shoulders are tense, that tension can pull on the fascia in your face, causing asymmetry, puffiness, and premature lines.

When Fascia & Muscle Tighten

1. **Tension imprints**
   From clenched jaws to furrowed brows, repeated expressions carve into your skin over time.
   Result *deep lines, sharp angles, heaviness in the lower face*

2. **Fascia pulls asymmetrically**
   We all have dominant sides and habits, like always chewing on one side. Over time, these create fascial imbalances that tug on the face unevenly.
   Result *facial asymmetry, uneven smile, or one eye sitting higher than the other*

3. **Muscles lock you in**
   Tight muscles overpower weaker ones, creating zones of activity or collapse.
   Result *sagging, compression, and loss of fluidity*

THE FASCIA-FACE CONNECTION IN ACTION

Problem	Symptoms
Jaw clenching	Compressed lower face
Head tension	Heavy brows and tired eyes
One-sided chewing	Facial asymmetry
Chronic frowning	Lasting forehead lines

Tight Fascia

Fascia functions like a web that covers your entire body, so when it becomes tight, dry, or scarred in one area, it can create tension and visible changes in other parts of the body, too.

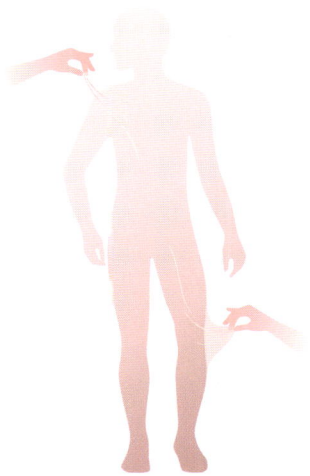

Key Players in Facial Fascia & Tension

Temporalis and occipital fascia
Head and scalp tension pull on the forehead and brows.

Frontalis
Constant lifting of the eyebrows locks forehead lines in place.

Masseter
One of the strongest muscles in your body. Chronic clenching can square the jaw and fold the skin.

Neck fascia
When tight, it tethers the lower face downwards.

The Muscles

Your face is home to over 40 unique muscles – delicate, expressive, and deeply interconnected. Unlike most body muscles, many facial muscles attach directly to the skin, allowing us to show emotion, speak, and shape our appearance. These illustrations reveal the key facial muscles involved in expression, aging, and facial mobility. Understanding their placement and function is the first step towards conscious connection and change. Whether you're lifting, releasing, or simply becoming aware, knowing what lies beneath your skin empowers every movement you make.

1. Galea aponeurotica
2. Frontalis
3. Temporalis
4. Procerus
5. Depressor supercili
6. Orbicularis oculi
7. Nasali (transverse portion)
8. Compressor narium minor
9. Dilator naris anterior
10. Nasalis (alar portion)
11. Levator labii superioris
12. Depressor septi nasi
13. Orbicularis oris
14. Levator labii superioris alaeque nasi
15. Zygomaticus minor
16. Levator anguli oris
17. Zygomaticus major
18. Modiolus
19. Masseter
20. Buccinator
21. Risorius
22. Depressor anguli oris
23. Depressor labii inferioris
24. Mentalis
25. Platysma

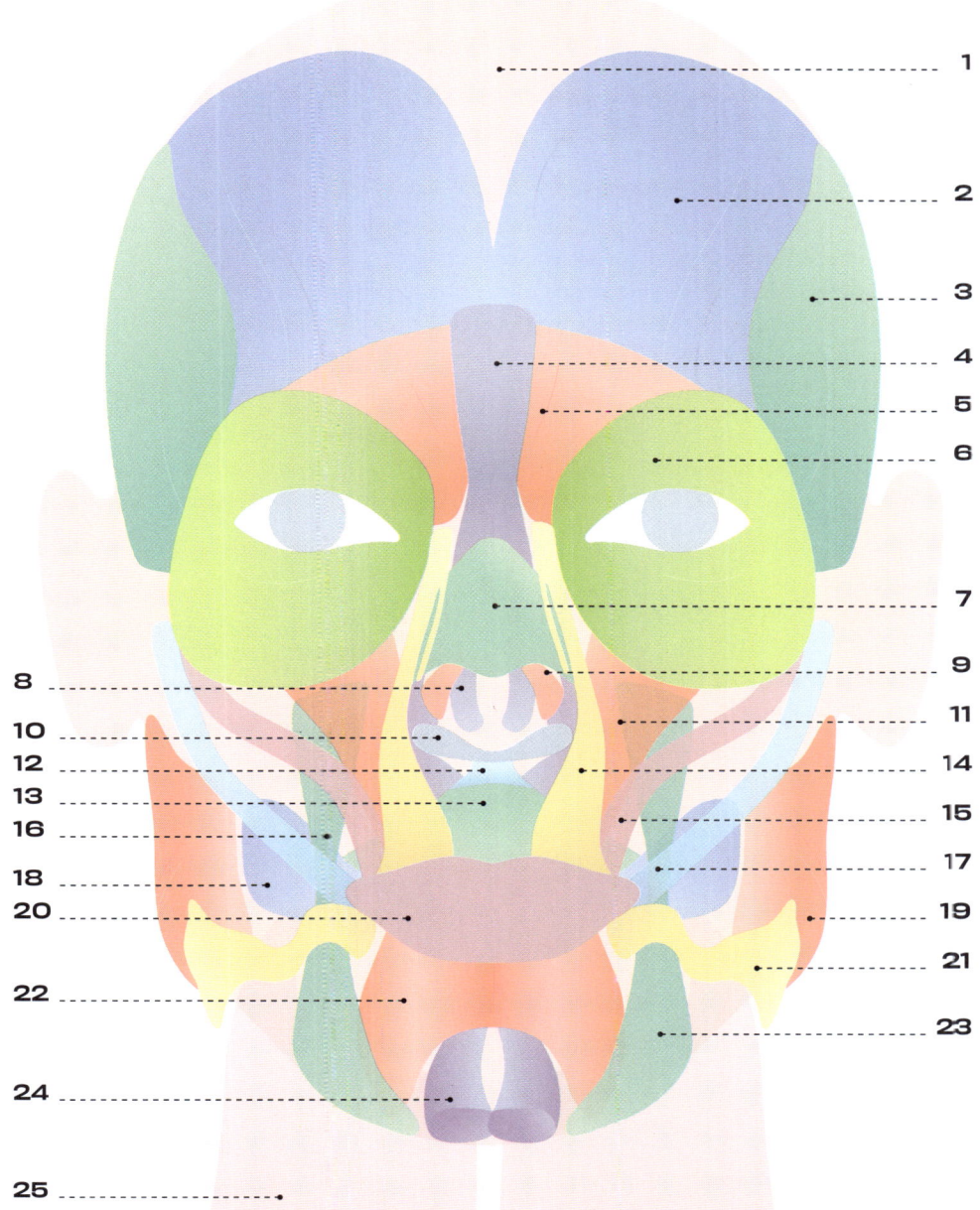

Loss of Muscle & Support

The Effects of Losing Support

Muscles aren't just for movement – they also provide support, shape, and lift to your face. But just like in the rest of the body, facial muscles can weaken or waste away if they're not used regularly or effectively. When this happens, the skin and fat lose their support structure.

Over time, if a muscle is chronically overused, it shortens, pulling the skin and reducing the surface area available. A wrinkle is the visible crease of a muscle that has lost flexibility.

When Muscles Are Underused

1. **Formation of wrinkles**
   Muscles that aren't stretched or moved become stiff and short, pulling the skin into creases.
   Result *static lines, especially on the forehead, between the brows, and around the mouth*

2. **Fat pads shrink**
   Loss of support from muscles and fascia can cause some fat pads to shrink while others may descend due to gravity.
   Result *under-eye hollows, jowls, and a sunken appearance*

3. **Loss of facial definition**
   The jawline blurs, cheeks flatten, and the mid-face drops.
   Result *sagging and loss of contour*

THE MUSCLE-FACE CONNECTION IN ACTION

Problem	Symptoms
Weak cheeks	Hollow under-eyes and saggy mid-face
Inactive jaw	Jowls and undefined jawline
Shortened muscles	Deep wrinkles and expression lines
Loss of tone	Tired, aged appearance

FACE YOGA

Key Players in Muscle Loss

1. **Orbicularis oculi**
   Weak tone leads to under-eye hollows and drooping lids.

2. **Zygomaticus major and minor**
   Underuse flattens the cheeks and diminishes natural lift.

3. **Buccinator and risorius**
   Loss of tone contributes to nasolabial folds and mouth sagging.

4. **Platysma**
   When inactive or overstretched, it loses its support function – leading to neck sag and jawline blur.

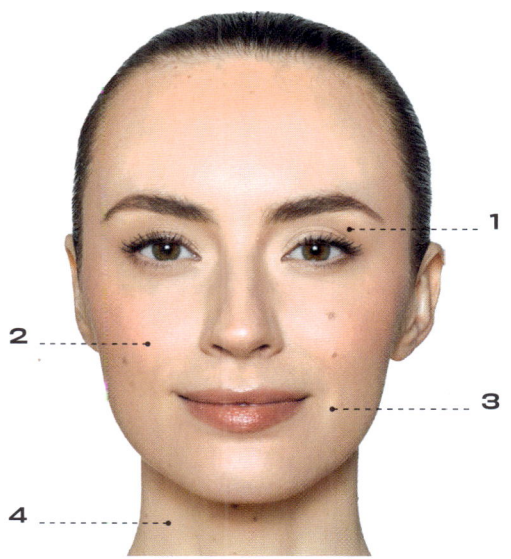

Losing Fat Pads

Superficial fat pads are responsible for facial curves and smooth transitions. Deep fat pads provide structural support closer to the bone and help maintain mid-face lift. When these fat pads shrink, areas of your face such as your cheeks and under-eyes begin to sag or hollow, and facial architecture starts to shift.

Youthful　　　　Aging

UNDERSTAND YOUR FACE

Tongue & Oral Posture

The Anatomy of Tongue Posture & Facial Form

Where your tongue rests shapes your entire mid-face and jawline. Your tongue acts as an internal support beam. When it sits high on the roof of the mouth and you breathe through your nose, it stimulates proper bone growth and supports facial symmetry.

But when the tongue sits low – or worse, when you breathe through your mouth – your facial muscles compensate. Your chin recedes. Your cheeks hollow. Your jaw weakens. And volume shifts down and out.

When Oral Posture is Off

1. **Midface weakens**
   Without the tongue supporting the palate, the upper jaw narrows and cheeks lose projection.
   Result *hollow cheeks, tired-looking eyes*

2. **Jawline loses definition**
   Mouth breathing alters muscle tone and increases fat deposition under the chin.
   Result *double chin, jawline blur*

3. **Facial structure slips**
   Tongue posture influences not just soft tissue, but bone remodelling over time.
   Result *imbalance, descent, and changes in nasal and oral shape*

THE TONGUE-FACE CONNECTION IN ACTION

Habit	Symptoms
Mouth breathing	Double chin and mid-face weakness
Low tongue posture	Flattened cheeks and jawline blur
Poor swallowing habits	Facial asymmetry and tension lines

WHAT IS MEWING — AND WHY IT MATTERS

The term "mewing" was popularized by Dr John Mew and Dr Mike Mew. Mewing refers to the conscious practice of placing the entire tongue flat against the roof of the mouth, lightly closing the lips, and breathing through the nose. The tongue is a postural muscle that helps shape the mid-face, palate, and jawline through constant, subtle pressure, so this posture supports the palate from within and can, over time, help improve facial structure, especially when adopted during younger developmental years.

Key Areas Affected by Tongue Posture

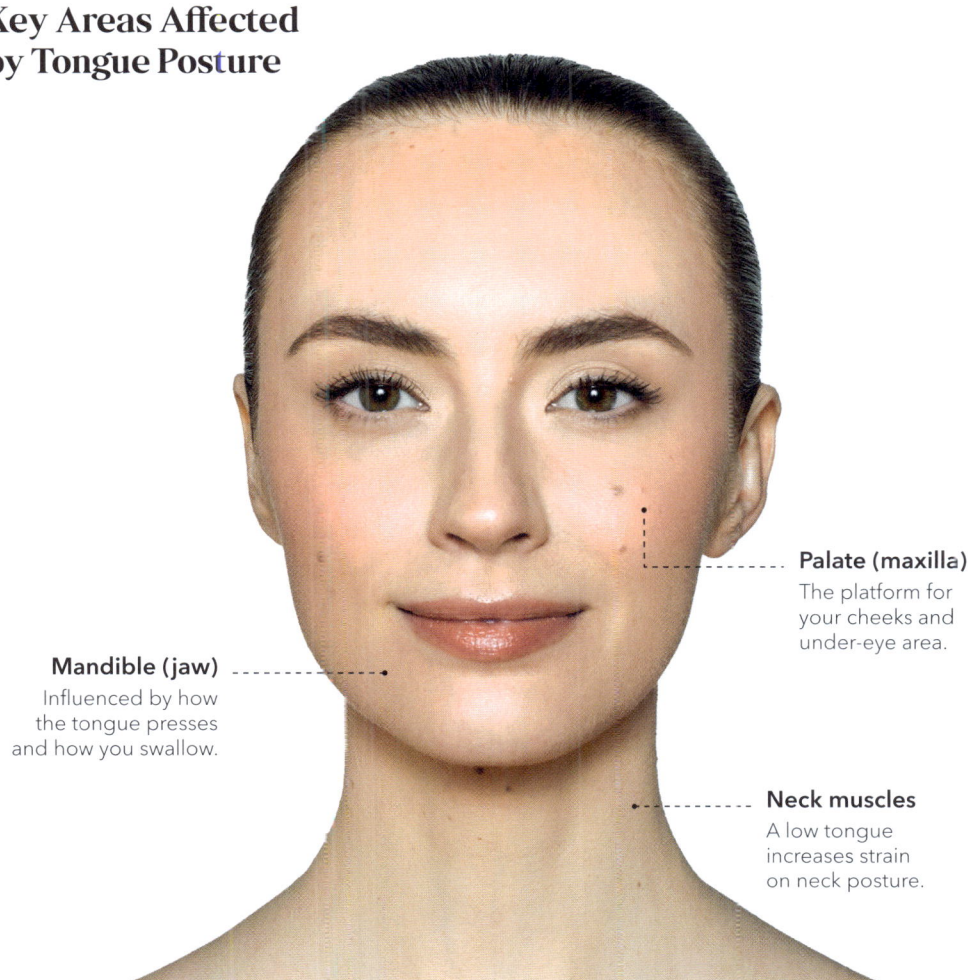

Palate (maxilla)
The platform for your cheeks and under-eye area.

Mandible (jaw)
Influenced by how the tongue presses and how you swallow.

Neck muscles
A low tongue increases strain on neck posture.

UNDERSTAND YOUR FACE

Lymphatic Stagnation

The Anatomy Behind Flow & Glow

Your skin is a living, breathing organ, but it can't thrive if it's not fed and cleaned from the inside. Your circulatory system delivers oxygen and nutrients to every skin cell. Your lymphatic system clears waste and stagnant fluid. But these systems rely on movement, breath, and open posture to work.

When we're emotionally closed, sedentary, or tense, blood and lymph flow can constrict. Over time, this contributes to many of the visible changes we associate with aging. However, when blood and lymph flow is strong, your skin glows.

When Flow Gets Blocked

1. **Lymph builds up**
   Tight muscles and slouched posture compress key drainage points, especially around your collarbones and neck.
   Result *puffiness, water retention, swollen eyes and jaw*

2. **Blood flow decreases**
   Shallow breath, clenching, and muscle tension restrict blood flow, like a crimped hose.
   Result *dull complexion, slower regeneration, lack of glow*

3. **Detox slows down**
   Without movement or breath, cellular waste builds up beneath the skin.
   Result *congestion, breakouts, and a tired, "dull" appearance*

THE LYMPHATIC-FACE CONNECTION IN ACTION

Problem	Symptoms
Neck tension	Puffy cheeks and jawline
Shallow breathing	Dull skin and toxin buildup
Compressed collarbone area	Swollen eyes and fluid retention

Key Flow Zones

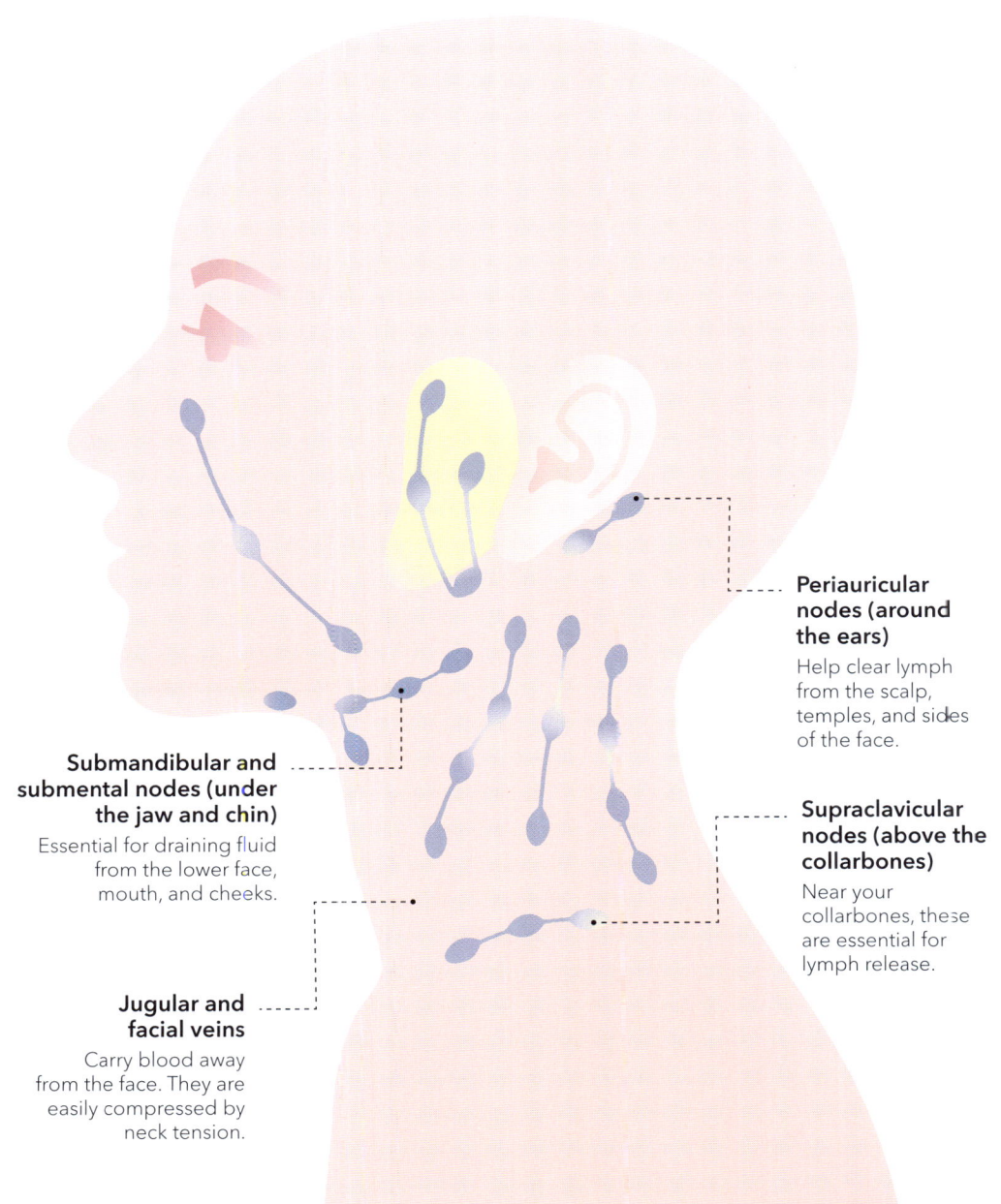

Periauricular nodes (around the ears)
Help clear lymph from the scalp, temples, and sides of the face.

Submandibular and submental nodes (under the jaw and chin)
Essential for draining fluid from the lower face, mouth, and cheeks.

Supraclavicular nodes (above the collarbones)
Near your collarbones, these are essential for lymph release.

Jugular and facial veins
Carry blood away from the face. They are easily compressed by neck tension.

UNDERSTAND YOUR FACE

The Lymphatic System

Your lymphatic system is your body's internal cleansing and recycling network. Unlike your circulatory system, which has the heart as a pump, lymph relies on muscle movement, posture, breath, and fascia elasticity to flow. Lymph clears cellular waste, filters toxins, and helps regulate fluid balance. But when flow stagnates – through tension, stillness, or poor alignment – your skin dulls, puffiness builds, and your body feels heavy and sluggish.

The good news? Simple daily movements and breath-led practices can reactivate this hidden highway, supporting both facial glow and whole-body vitality.

When Lymph Flow Stalls

1 **Stillness slows the pump**
   Without muscle contraction, lymph fluid pools. Long hours of sitting or shallow breathing rob the system of its natural momentum.
   Result *heavy legs, swollen hands, puffy face*

2 **Postural compression blocks drainage**
   Slouched posture collapses lymphatic exit points (such as the collarbones and groin), creating a bottleneck.
   Result *fluid retention, swelling, and sluggish detox*

3 **Tense fascia restricts pathways**
   Sticky fascia binds lymph vessels, making it harder for fluid to move freely.
   Result *congestion, uneven tone, visible puffiness*

THE LYMPH–BODY CONNECTION IN ACTION

Problem	Symptoms
Neck tension	Blocked facial drainage and puffy jawline
Collapsed chest	Fluid pooling in the face and hands
Sluggish legs	Tired, heavy feeling and reduced glow

Key Lymphatic Highways

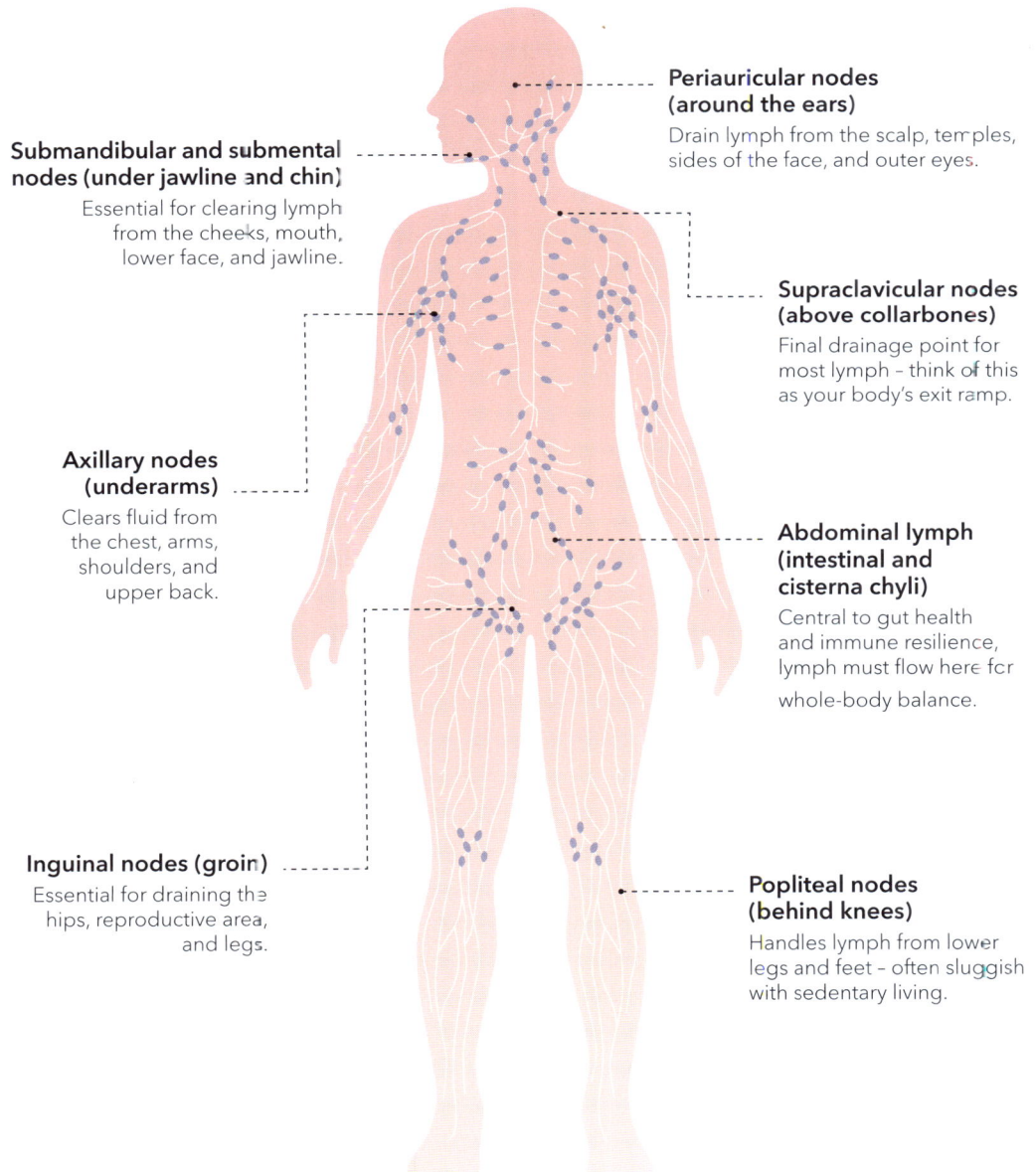

Submandibular and submental nodes (under jawline and chin)
Essential for clearing lymph from the cheeks, mouth, lower face, and jawline.

Axillary nodes (underarms)
Clears fluid from the chest, arms, shoulders, and upper back.

Inguinal nodes (groin)
Essential for draining the hips, reproductive area, and legs.

Periauricular nodes (around the ears)
Drain lymph from the scalp, temples, sides of the face, and outer eyes.

Supraclavicular nodes (above collarbones)
Final drainage point for most lymph – think of this as your body's exit ramp.

Abdominal lymph (intestinal and cisterna chyli)
Central to gut health and immune resilience, lymph must flow here for whole-body balance.

Popliteal nodes (behind knees)
Handles lymph from lower legs and feet – often sluggish with sedentary living.

UNDERSTAND YOUR FACE

Emotional Holding Patterns
The Anatomy of Expression & Emotion

Your face is the canvas of your emotional life. But what happens when emotions get stuck, or never get fully expressed? Micro-holdings – those tiny, unconscious contractions in our muscles – become macro patterns over time.

What starts as a barely perceptible clench in the jaw, furrow in the brow, or tightness around the mouth can, when repeated daily, etch itself into the face as a permanent expression. These micro-holdings act like emotional fingerprints, quietly sculpting the features into long-term patterns that reflect how we've carried stress or emotion over the years.

3 Emotional fatigue
When we can't express, we suppress. That suppression often lives in the face. **Result** *lowered energy, slouched posture, or a chronically tired look*

When Emotions Take Up Residence

1 Chronic contraction
Clenched jaws, furrowed brows, and pursed lips become default settings. **Result** *static lines, locked features, and a face that doesn't match how you feel inside*

2 Protective postures
Stress and trauma often express through the muscles of the face and neck. **Result** *a shielded face – one that holds back softness, connection, or vulnerability*

THE EMOTIONS–FACE CONNECTION IN ACTION

Emotion	Symptoms
Unexpressed grief	Downturned mouth and hollowed eyes
Chronic stress	Furrowed brow and jaw clenching
Over-control	Tension around lips and eyes

FACE YOGA

Key Muscle-Emotion Connections

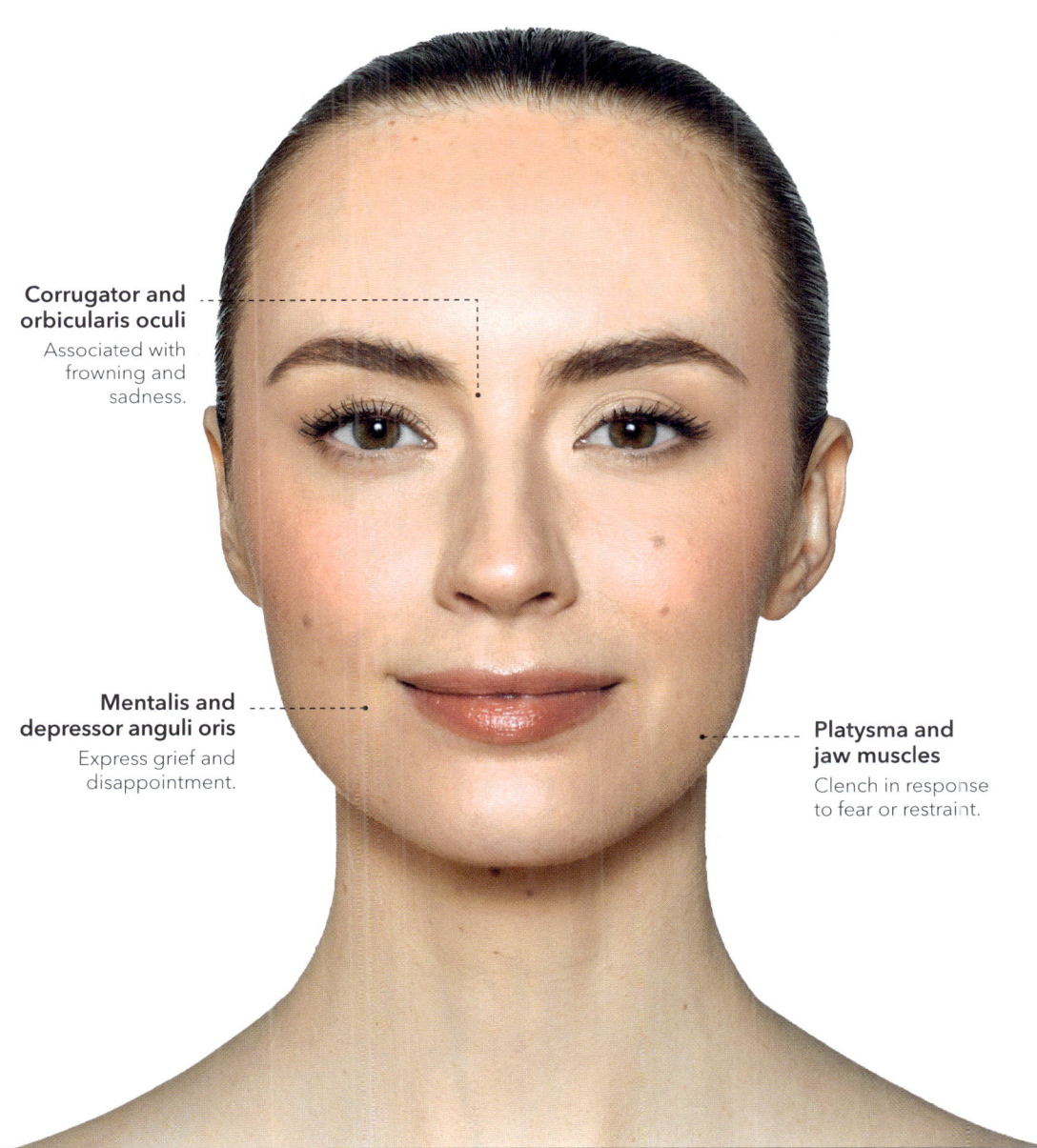

Corrugator and orbicularis oculi
Associated with frowning and sadness.

Mentalis and depressor anguli oris
Express grief and disappointment.

Platysma and jaw muscles
Clench in response to fear or restraint.

Structural Remodelling
The Anatomy of Facial Bones

The facial skeleton is not static; over time, it naturally remodels, reshapes, and gradually shrinks, which is known as bone resorption. This resorption reduces the support for soft tissues such as fat, muscles, and skin, causing them to shift, descend, or fold.

But this isn't just caused by genetics or time. Lifestyle plays a huge role. Think of it like muscle weakness, but in your bone tissue. Without consistent mechanical load from movement, posture, and muscle engagement, the facial framework can begin to shrink or collapse inwards, leading to the skin sinking in, hollowing of the cheeks or temples, and an overall loss of facial support.

What Accelerates Bone Remodelling

1. **Lack of muscle engagement**
   Without healthy muscle tension, bone density declines.
   Result *volume loss, collapsing structure, shifting fat pads*

2. **Poor posture and alignment**
   Chronically compressed cervical spine alters the facial bone structure over time.
   Result *jaw recession, changes to the bite and facial profile*

3. **Nutrient deficiencies**
   Low levels of calcium, magnesium, and vitamin D slow bone repair.
   Result *fragility, sunken features*

THE BONE-FACE CONNECTION IN ACTION

Problem	Symptoms
Receding jaw	Weakened profile and sagging skin
Flattened cheekbones	Mid-face collapse
Bone loss	Hollow temples and under-eye shadow

Bone Resorption

Just like the hips or spine, facial bones are subject to bone density loss over time – especially when underused.

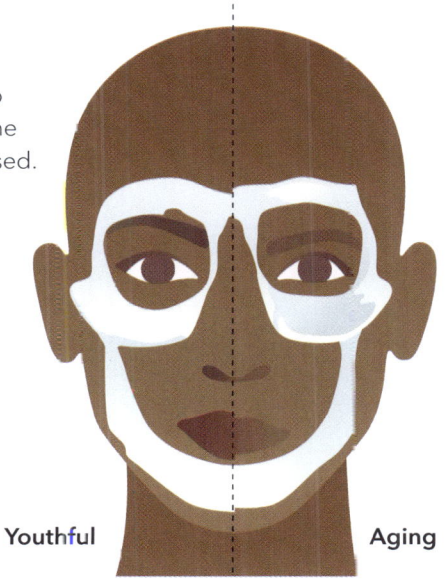

Youthful   Aging

Key Bone Structures that Shape the Face

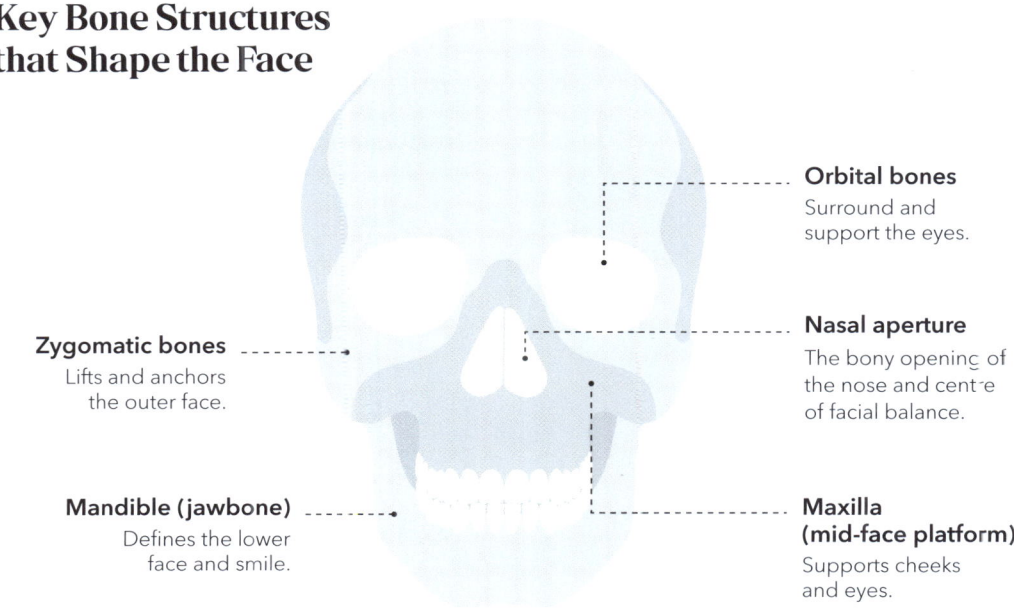

Zygomatic bones
Lifts and anchors the outer face.

Mandible (jawbone)
Defines the lower face and smile.

Orbital bones
Surround and support the eyes.

Nasal aperture
The bony opening of the nose and centre of facial balance.

Maxilla (mid-face platform)
Supports cheeks and eyes.

UNDERSTAND YOUR FACE

Lifestyle Rhythms & Cellular Stress

The Physiology of Modern Aging

It's not just time that ages us; it's how we spend that time. From artificial light to ultra-processed food, to the media we consume and the people we surround ourselves with, modern living sends conflicting signals to our biology. Chronic stress, emotional tension, digital overload, and even toxic relationships can all manifest visibly on the face, amplifying signs of aging.

When Daily Life Wears You Down

1. **Inflammation increases**
   Stress, sugar, and lack of sleep promote cellular damage.
   Result *slower collagen repair, more visible aging*

2. **Glycation and oxidation**
   Glycation occurs when excess sugar in the bloodstream binds to proteins, forming molecules called Advanced Glycation End-products (AGEs), which damage collagen and elastin, making skin less supple and more prone to sagging and wrinkles.
   Result *sagging, uneven tone, poor elasticity*

3. **Circadian disruption**
   Late nights and screen exposure confuse the body's repair rhythms.
   Result *tired eyes, poor skin texture, slowed regeneration*

THE LIFESTYLE-FACE CONNECTION IN ACTION

Posture	Symptoms
Poor sleep	Dark circles and puffy eyes
Excess sugar	Sagging skin and uneven tone
Chronic screen use	Tech neck and fatigued features

Key Lifestyle Influencers

Sleep and circadian rhythm
Skin regenerates at night. Rest is non-negotiable.

Breathing and nervous system
Shallow breath = chronic stress mode.

Diet and hydration
You literally become what you absorb.

Movement and physical activity
Regular movement improves circulation, oxygen delivery, and lymphatic flow.

Sunlight and nature exposure
Too little natural light or excessive artificial/indoor living leads to disrupted sleep, dull skin, and mood imbalance.

Toxins and environmental load
Air quality, pollution, smoking, and chemical exposure all influence oxidative stress and cellular aging.

Social connection and relationships
Supportive relationships lower cortisol, increase oxytocin, and foster resilience.

Mental and emotional landscape
Mindset, purpose, and emotional regulation shape how the nervous system operates daily.

Recovery and restorative practices
Stretching, fascia release, meditation, sauna, and cold exposure promote resilience and cellular repair.

Your Face Map
Discover Yourself From a New Perspective

The following exercise will help you observe yourself clearly, compassionately, and without filters. When you learn how to decode what you see, you can begin to work with your face as a partner – not a problem.

1 Scalp
Notice tension or tightness. A relaxed scalp lifts the whole face.

2 Forehead
Notice tens on, lines, and skin texture.

3 Eyebrows
Check for asymmetry, tension, or drooping.

4 Eyes
Observe puffiness, dark circles, fine lines, or asymmetry.

5 Cheeks
Check for volume loss, sagging, or tension.

6 Nose
Notice any tension, flaring, or widening. Is the shape relaxed or strained?

7 Nasolabial Folds
Notice the depth of the lines from nose to mouth. Are they pronounced or relaxed?

8 Mouth and Lips
Observe expression lines, drooping corners, or dryness.

9 Jawline
Look for tightness, jaw clenching, or lack of definition.

10 Neck
Check for tension, horizontal lines, or loose skin.

11 Collarbones
Are they open and relaxed or tense and rounded? Check your posture.

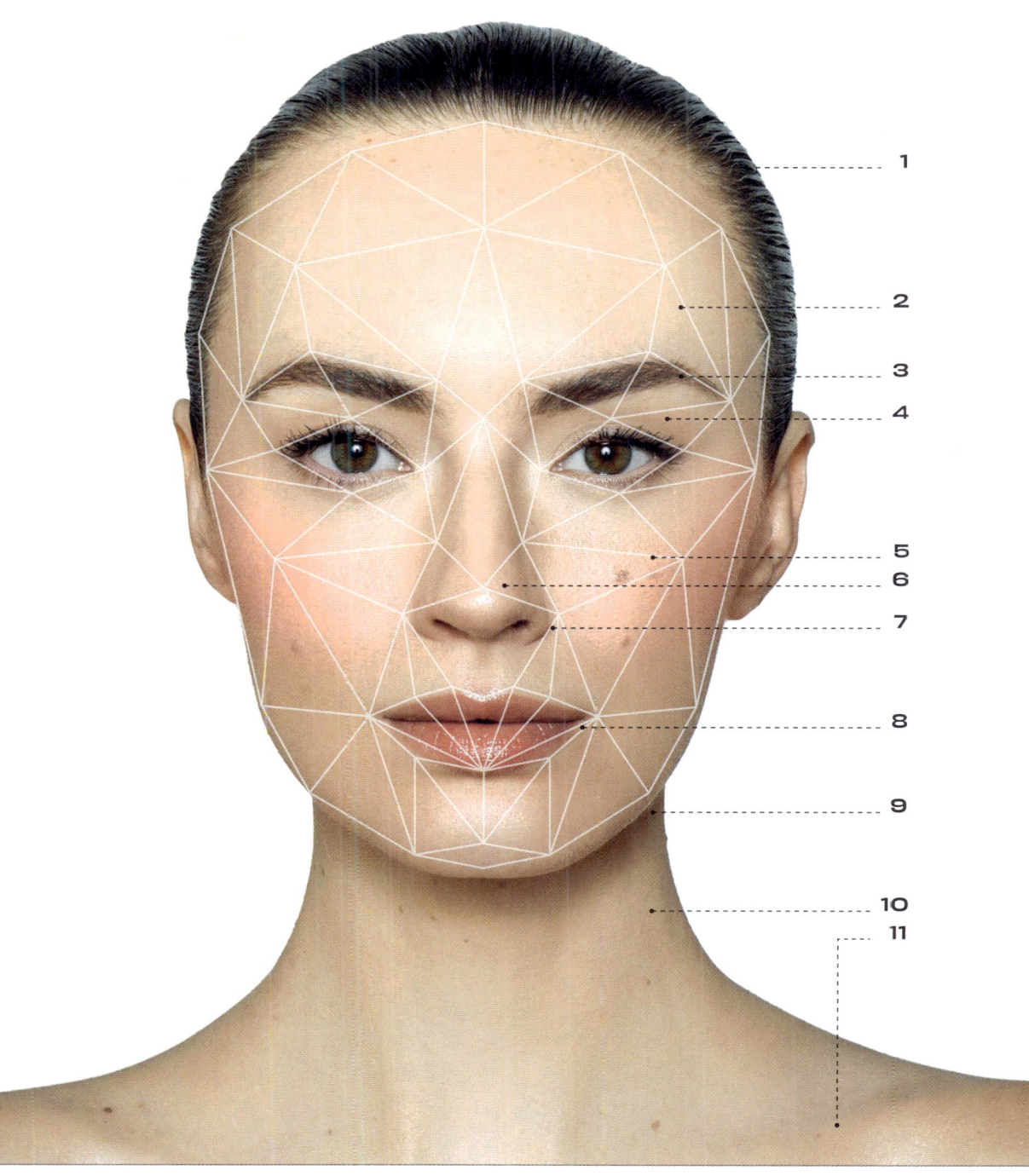

UNDERSTAND YOUR FACE

Self-Analyse Your Face

Learning to Observe Without Judgement

Just as a chiropractor reads your spine or a therapist tunes in to your tone of voice, this is your invitation to learn how to see your face beyond the surface. This is your opportunity to decode not just what you see – but what it might mean.

When you begin to notice the way one cheek lifts higher than the other, or how a line deepens more on one side of your mouth, you're not just spotting asymmetry. You're uncovering patterns: of posture, of movement, of emotion. These patterns tell a story – a story of habits, of holding, of protection.

You're not trying to change anything with this exercise just yet. You're simply gathering data, ready to explore the exercises and methods in Part 2 of this book.

Your Personal Facial Map

Start by standing in front of a mirror with soft, natural light. This isn't about performing or criticizing; it's about observing. Let yourself settle, and notice how your face looks when it's not "on". As you carry out this exercise, make a mental or physical note of your findings for each section.

Now, begin scanning your face gently, from scalp to collarbones. As you observe each area, feel free to mark down visual signs, but also go deeper. Pay attention to sensation. Use the pads of your fingers to gently press, pause, and feel beneath the surface – not just the skin, but the layers of fascia and muscle. Try small circles or side-to-side movements to detect tension or areas that feel dense or stuck. You can rate each area on a scale of 1 to 5, with 1 being not painful or tense at all, and 5 being extremely tender, tight, or uncomfortable. This scale will help you identify areas of holding or imbalance even if they don't show up visibly.

Side profile

Next, take a moment to assess your profile view. Turn to the side or use a second mirror to observe your profile. Is your head stacked in alignment over your shoulders, or does it jut forward? Is your chin level or tilted down? Look at the base of your neck. Does it have a visible hump or curve developed? This "tech neck" posture can compress vital lymph and blood flow pathways and may contribute to jaw tension, puffiness, and lower face sagging. Your profile tells a powerful part of the story, and often reveals more than we can see from the front.

Scalp

Is there tension at your crown or tightness where your hair meets the forehead? Do you often feel heat, pressure, or numbness in this area? Try moving the scalp with your fingertips – does it glide, or feel stuck and immobile? A healthy scalp has elasticity and mobility. If it feels puffy, congested, or fixed in place, it may signal fascial restrictions or stagnant lymph flow beneath the surface.

Forehead and brows

Are your brows level or does one sit higher? Is your forehead relaxed or etched with tension? Do you frequently raise your brows, even at rest? Press your fingertips against the skin. How does it feel? Check the elasticity. Is the skin easily lifted and moved, or does it feel stuck or tightly tethered to the skull? Does it bounce back when you release it, or stay creased? A mobile, responsive forehead often reflects hydration and healthy fascia; a stuck, rigid surface may point to underlying restriction or stress. Look also for pigmentation differences or uneven texture that may indicate longer-term stagnation or tension. Does the skin bounce back when you lift it, or does it feel rigid or slow to recover? Look for signs of dehydration, dullness, or pigmentation differences that may indicate stress or stagnation in circulation.

Eyes

Are your eyes open, bright, and soft, or do they squint or appear tired? Is one more lifted or drooping? Notice the skin texture and any puffiness or hollowness. If you see dark circles under your eyes, do this test: gently pinch the skin just below the eyes and observe the colour. If the darkness fades when the skin is lifted and then returns gradually, it may point to poor blood circulation or lymph stagnation. If the skin remains dark even when lifted, it's more likely due to deeper pigmentation or genetic factors, and may respond better to internal detox support, sun protection, and skin-brightening approaches. This simple test offers valuable insight into what your under-eye area might truly need.

Also check for crow's feet or fine lines at the outer corners of the eyes. These can often be signs of dehydration or overused orbicularis oculi muscles. Lightly stretch the area – does the skin feel papery, or does it glide smoothly? This can tell you a lot about hydration levels and where the muscles might need softening or support.

Nose

Does your nose sit centred or slightly tilted? Do you breathe freely through both nostrils, or is one side more dominant? Use your fingertips to gently feel around the sides and bridge of the nose. Do you notice tension in the surrounding muscles, or does the area feel soft and mobile? Chronic scrunching or tightness here can create asymmetries, widen the bridge, or affect the way you breathe and express. Tension in this area may also subtly influence the positioning of the brows, eyes, and upper lip.

Cheeks and nasolabial folds

Are your cheeks lifted or flat? Do both sides match in fullness? Are your nasolabial lines (the lines that run from the sides of your nostrils to the corners of your mouth) even or deeper on one side? This can reveal muscle dominance or structural support loss. Gently touch your cheeks with your fingertips. Do the muscles feel soft and responsive, or do you detect areas of tension or tightness? Tension in the zygomatic or buccinator muscles (see page 18) can contribute to restricted movement, asymmetry, or even premature folds in this region. Also notice the connection between your cheeks and your lower eyelids. Is there a visible crease, line, or sense of pulling between these areas? This can indicate accumulated tension that affects both zones and may need to be released together.

Mouth and lips

Is your mouth relaxed or subtly pursed? Are your lips full and hydrated, or dry and tense? Notice if one side of the mouth pulls more when you speak or smile. Try gently grabbing your lips between your thumb and index finger. Do you feel tightness, especially at the corners of the mouth? This area is where multiple muscle strands from the cheeks and mouth converge. Tension here may indicate emotional holding, clenching habits, or imbalance in muscle use. Also check for symmetry. Do the corners of the mouth sit evenly or is one slightly lower or pulled outwards? This can reflect imbalances in muscle tone or habitual movement patterns that affect how your expressions form and settle.

Jawline

Is there visible clenching or tension along the masseter? (see page 18) Is your jaw more defined on one side? Check for asymmetry or tightness. Try opening your mouth gently and pressing along the sides of your jaw – do you feel tenderness, resistance, or muscle guarding? You can also do the four-finger test: can you comfortably fit your index to pinky finger (held together vertically) inside your mouth when it's open? If not, this may indicate muscular restriction or joint tension in the temporomandibular joint (TMJ) area, which are the joints that connect your skull to your lower jaw on each side of your head, in front of your ears.

Neck and SCM (Sternocleidomastoid)

Is your neck long and relaxed or compressed? Run your fingers along the SCM (the ropey muscle from behind the ear to the collarbone, see page 18). Is one side more rigid or tender? Try gently grabbing the muscle between your fingers. Does it feel soft and elastic, or do you experience pain, tightness, or resistance? Pain or tenderness here can signal stored tension, restricted circulation, or postural strain.

Collarbone and upper chest

Are your collarbones visible and lifted, or sunken and compressed? Do you feel breath move easily through your chest, or is it shallow? Check the position of your collarbones. Are they sitting relatively horizontal and symmetrical, or are they slanted unevenly or pulled upwards? When the collarbones are collapsed or compressed, they can press into vital pathways, restricting blood and lymph flow from the head, face, and neck. Proper collarbone positioning supports clear circulation and fluid drainage, which is essential for facial tone and glow.

Tension points

Where do you instinctively touch or rub your face and neck? Common tension zones include the temples, jaw hinge, cheeks, and base of the skull. These are your holding patterns.

> **BONUS CHECK-IN: GRAVITY TEST**
>
> *Hold a mirror in front of your face, then slowly tilt your head forwards so it's parallel to the floor. Watch closely: which areas begin to droop or shift downwards first? These are often the earliest signs of facial changes. They may be subtle, but they tend to deepen over time. Awareness is the first step towards change.*

THE METHOD & MOVEMENTS

The All You Can Face Method

Your Face Tells Your Story

The All You Can Face Method is more than a series of exercises. It's a modern, science-backed approach to reconnecting with your facial structure, reclaiming your expression, and reactivating deep layers of tissue that often got neglected in traditional beauty routines. It blends ancient wisdom, modern anatomy, and emotional awareness into a powerful daily ritual that restores both appearance and inner presence.

Most of us train our bodies but forget that the face, too, is made of muscles, many of which are under conscious control and responsive to training. But unlike the rest of the body, facial muscles are uniquely delicate. They sit just beneath the skin and often attach to other muscles or soft tissue rather than bones. This makes them incredibly expressive but also highly susceptible to tension, stagnation, and collapse if left inactive or overused.

Think of your face as a system – not a surface. Every muscle, every line, every expression is connected to how you sit, breathe, think, and feel. That's why this method doesn't stop at surface sculpting. It targets deep, intentional layers, helping you create lasting change from within.

True transformation starts with conscious observation. Before you begin to move, you learn to see, as we have done in the first part of this book. This builds anatomical awareness and invites you to analyse your unique facial structure, habits, and imbalances. It's about understanding with what's really going on under the skin.

The method then follows three distinct and interwoven phases:

1

Posture Practice
Your face is deeply influenced by the alignment of your neck, spine, and shoulders. In this first phase, you reset your posture to build a stable foundation, as when your body is aligned, facial work becomes more effective and sustainable.

2

Release Tension
This phase targets areas of chronic tightness and overuse – from clenched jaws and furrowed brows to stiff necks and locked shoulders. Gentle stretches and fascia release techniques help to melt away tension and stagnation, creating more space and flow in your tissues.

3

Strengthen
Now, you rebuild. This phase reawakens underused muscles, especially those responsible for lifting, support, and expression. With focused, low-resistance exercises, you bring strength and vitality back to your face, naturally sculpting your features and refreshing your appearance from the inside out.

Each movement has a holistic focus, which goes far beyond aesthetics. Releasing the jaw can improve sleep. Lifting the cheeks can boost your mood. Restoring facial mobility supports healthy aging and deeper self-connection.

You don't need hours in front of the mirror. Most routines take under 10 minutes and can be adapted to your needs – energize in the morning, reset in the afternoon, and unwind before bed.

As you begin this journey, remember: it's not just about looking better. It's about feeling better. More alive, more confident, more *you*.

Let's begin.

How to Build Your Routine

Creating Your Personalized Routine

So far, you've taken the time to observe your face, and to understand what's really going on beneath your skin. Now it's time to take these observations and use them, and the exercises in the following chapter, to build your own personal face yoga routines. The movements in this book are best practised as part of a routine, so follow the guidelines below to build your own.

To begin building your own routines:

1 Identify what area(s) to focus on
Are their any specific concerns you want to address? Each exercise details which part of the face it works with, and the effects the movement has when practised consistently.

2 Decide on the length of your routine
Each exercise includes a time or repetitions shortcut icon so that you can see how long each move is going to take. Don't forget to factor in some rest time between each exercise (see page 46).

3 Choose your exercises
Read through the exercises in this chapter and choose ones that align with your goals, and will fit into your schedule.

4 Structure your routine
Use the advice below to structure your routine in the most effective order.

5 Track your progress
Use a notebook or app to map your goals and track your progress. Remember that the goal is not perfection – it's consistency.

You can create a new ritual for each day, or create one routine each week, to be practised daily.
  Whether you're practising for 5 or 15 minutes, remember: it's about reconnecting with yourself, step by step.

Follow the 3-Phase System

This chapter is separated into three key phases, and when building your routine, it is helpful to structure your exercises following this order to set you up for lasting results.

Phase 1 Posture Practice
Start with posture to establish a sturdy foundation.

Phase 2 Release Tension
Release tension to create space.

Phase 3 Strengthen
Strengthen with awareness and control.

Icons Key

Each exercise includes an icon to show you which area of the face or technique it addresses. Whether you're working on puffiness, asymmetry, wrinkles, or muscle tone, these will help guide your choices.

 Lymphatic system activity

 Posture activity

 Massage activity

 Upper face

 Lower face

HOW TO BALANCE YOUR ROUTINE

When developing your own routines, whether it's a quick five-minute boost, or a longer session, it's helpful to follow the following formula:

30% Phase 1 exercises | 30% Phase 2 exercises | 40% Phase 3 exercises

Before You Begin
How to Get Started

Before you begin your routines, take a moment to centre yourself. This journey is about understanding your face, your body, and your inner voice – not about chasing perfection.

The following guidelines will help you build a safe, effective, and sustainable practice.

DO

+ **Start with clean hands and a clean face** Before beginning any face training, make sure your hands are freshly washed and your face is free of makeup or residue. This keeps your skin clear, prevents breakouts, and helps make your touch more sensitive and intentional.

+ **Relax between exercises** The moments of rest between each exercise are as valuable as the movements themselves. They allow your muscles, fascia, and nervous system to integrate what you've done.

+ **Maintain good posture throughout** When practising any exercises, begin by sitting or stand tall with your feet hip-width apart. Distribute your weight evenly, soften your knees and relax your shoulders and face. Open your chest, breathe deeply through your nose, and let your face relax. Keep your spine tall, shoulders relaxed, and chest open.

+ **Take your time** Rushing through the exercises won't serve you. Attention and presence lead to better results.

DO	DON'T
+ **Check yourself in a mirror** The mirror is your best teacher, especially at the beginning of your face yoga journey, as it ensures you're using the correct muscles without creating unwanted tension or wrinkles elsewhere.	+ **Don't ignore pain** Mild tenderness is normal as you awaken new muscles and release tension. But if you feel sharp pain or nerve discomfort, stop. Recheck the instructions before continuing.
+ **Practise on both sides** Symmetry is a core principle of facial harmony. It's okay to focus a little more on the side that feels weaker or looks less balanced, but aim for overall evenness.	+ **Don't overdo it** More is not always better. These exercises are powerful. Practise in moderation, always combining strengthening with release to maintain balance.
+ **Visualize the muscles you're working** The mind-body connection is powerful. Even when a movement feels subtle or difficult, intentional focus will help.	+ **Don't create unwanted wrinkles** If you notice creases forming in other areas (for example, frowning while working your under-eyes), slow down or gently support those areas with your fingers.
+ **Moisturize if needed** If your skin feels dry, apply a light cream or oil. This protects your skin from unnecessary stretching while you work. I'll advise if there are any exercises where oil is mandatory.	+ **Don't hold your breath** Keep your breathing soft and steady. Breath fuels your practice and calms your nervous system.
+ **Time lymphatic techniques wisely** These are best done at least 2-3 hours before bedtime, as they can stimulate circulation and energy flow – not ideal when you're preparing for rest.	+ **Don't pull or tug the skin** This method builds from the inside out – working with your muscles as the foundation for your skin's support.
	+ **Don't repeat the same pose excessively** Variation matters. Muscles, like any part of your body, need both work and rest.

PHASE 01
POSTURE PRACTICE

Before we touch a single facial muscle, we begin where true transformation starts: with your posture. Your face is part of a dynamic system, deeply connected to your neck, spine, shoulders, and chest. When these areas collapse – from tech neck, daily stress, or old habits – your facial structure follows.

In this phase, you'll learn how to align your body to give your face the support it needs. You'll unlock tension in your neck, open your chest, and create space for blood, oxygen, and lymph to flow freely to your skin and muscles.

This is the foundation of everything that comes next. Without it, any face work will have limited impact, because true facial vitality begins with your posture.

The Lymphatic Assessment 50
The Big 6 Lymphatic Activation 52
100 Jumps 54
The Neck Tap 55
The Shoulder Warm-Up 56
The Neck Warm-Up 57
The Neck Stretch 58
The Knuckle Rotation 59
The Ballerina Neck 60
The Heart Opener Stretch 61
The Shoulder Hug Stretch 62
The Diagonal Neck Release 63
The Angel Wings 64
The Armpit & Arm Opener 65
The Shoulder Realigner 66
The Standing Chest Stretch 67
The Wall Side Stretch 68
The Standing Chest Glide 69
Wall Shoulder Chest Opener 70
The Neck Reset 71
The Shoulder Spiral 72
The Neck Resistance Press 73

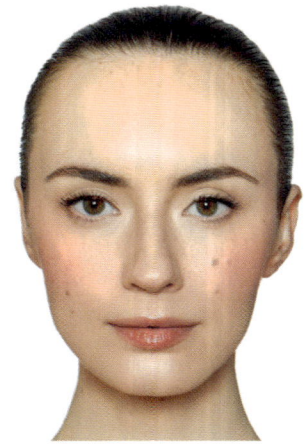
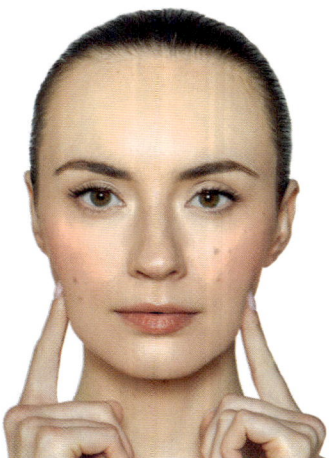
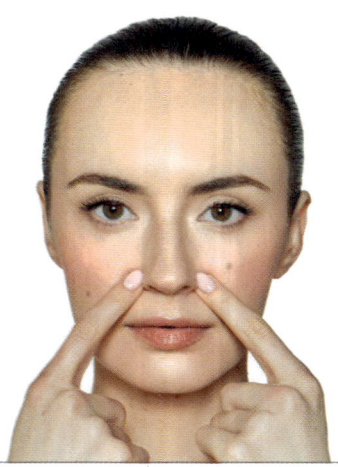

 1–2 MIN

The Lymphatic Assessment

Check in with your face

Before diving into drainage techniques, it's helpful to assess whether your lymphatic system is sluggish or blocked. By gently pressing on specific facial drainage points, you can identify areas of stagnation, puffiness, or tenderness, which are all subtle signals that your system needs support.

1 **Check key points**
Using the pads of your fingers, gently press on the following lymphatic checkpoints:

+ **Along your jawline,** especially near the centre of the chin and under the ears

+ **Beside your nostrils,** on the soft tissue to either side of your nose

+ **At the outer edge of your eyebrows,** just beyond the temple area

+ **Behind the angle of your jaw,** where your neck meets your jawline (under the earlobe)

FACE YOGA

2 Notice tenderness
Apply light to medium pressure. If these areas feel puffy, tender, congested, or sensitive, it may be a sign that your lymphatic system is not draining efficiently. This is especially common in times of stress, illness, travel, or lack of movement.

3 Use it as a guide
Let what you feel guide what exercises you choose to do next. Areas of tenderness can benefit most from gentle drainage, fascia release, or breath-led relaxation.

> **TIP**
> This check-in is not about judgement; it's about supporting your system where it needs it most. You can repeat this assessment weekly to track changes and progress over time.

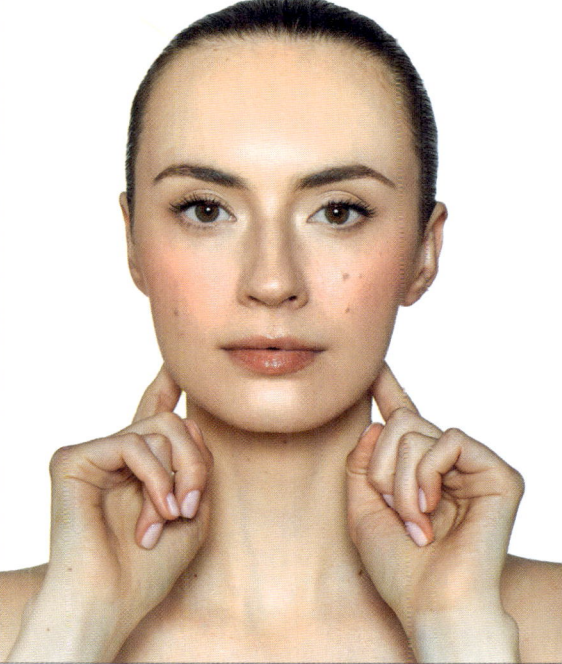

THE METHOD & MOVEMENTS | 51

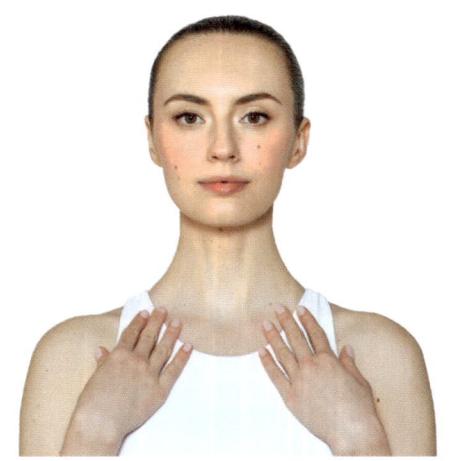
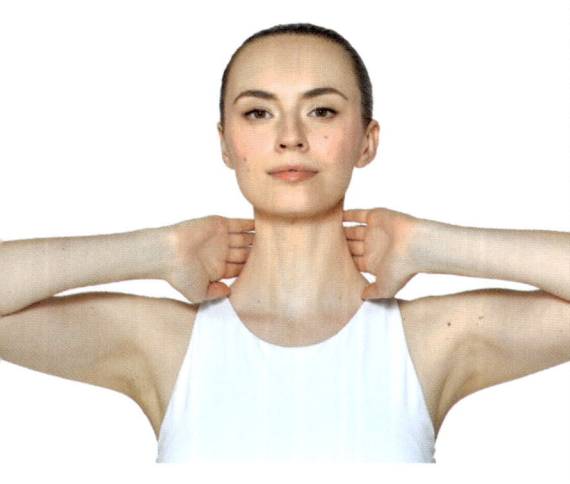
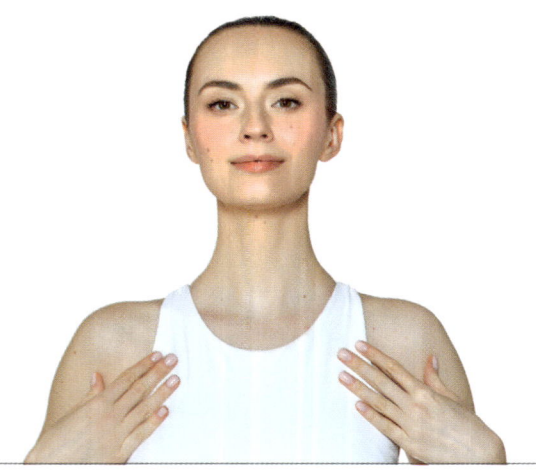

 4.5 MIN

The Big 6 Lymphatic Activation

Encourage your whole system to flow freely

Based on Dr Perry Nickelston's "Big 6" method, this sequence stimulates your body's primary lymphatic drainage points. Do this sequence before any facial work or movement, as long as it's not too close to bedtime (see page 47).

1 **Massage your collarbones (supraclavicular area)**
Gently tap or massage in small circles above your collarbones for 30 seconds. This is the final drainage site for most lymph in the body.

2 **Stroke your neck (jugular and cervical nodes)**
Using light brushing motions with your fingertips, stroke downwards from just below your ears to your collarbones. Do this for 30 seconds on each side to help move lymph from the face, scalp, and head into the collarbone drainage zone.

3 **Massage your underarms (axillary nodes)**
Massage your armpits using small circles or open-handed tapping for 30 seconds on each side to clear drainage from the chest, shoulders, arms, and breasts.

4 **Massage your belly
(abdominal / intestinal lymph)**
Massage the soft area just inside and below your ribs with circular, clockwise motions for 30 seconds, breathing deeply into your abdomen. This area is central to digestive flow and gut-based immune support.

5 **Massage your groin (inguinal nodes)**
Press gently into the groin area and massage in small circles for 30 seconds to clear lymph from the legs, hips, and reproductive organs.

6 **Massage your knees (popliteal nodes)**
Gently massage behind each knee for 30 seconds on each side to drain lymph from your lower legs and feet.

WHY THE ORDER MATTERS

Your lymphatic system works like gravity-fed plumbing: it needs clear exit points to flow. That's why we start at the collarbones, the final face drainage site, and work our way back up, and then down through the system. If you stimulate the limbs or face first, but your exits are blocked, the lymph has nowhere to go, causing more congestion, not less.

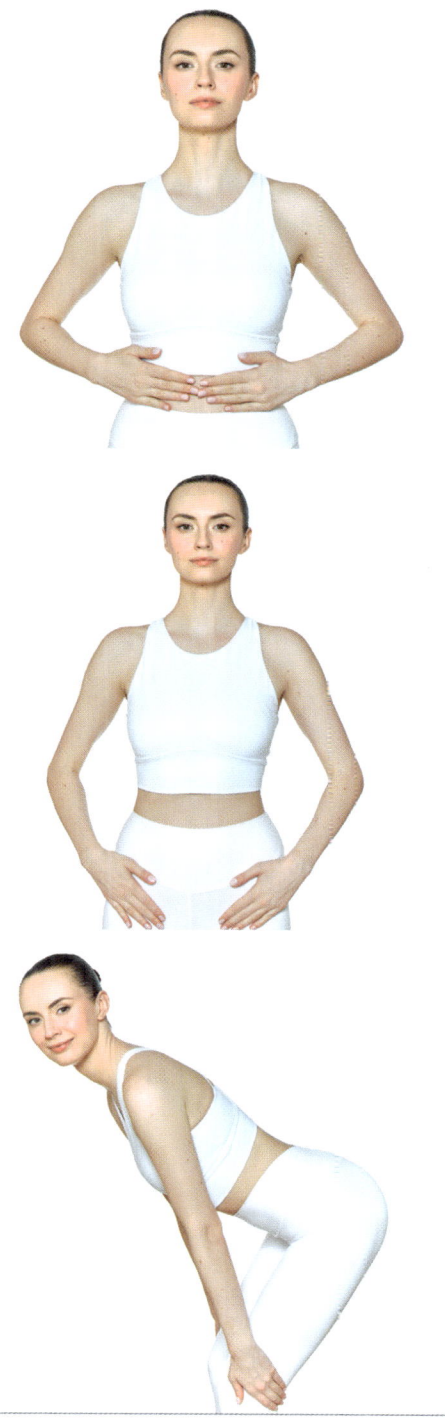

THE METHOD & MOVEMENTS

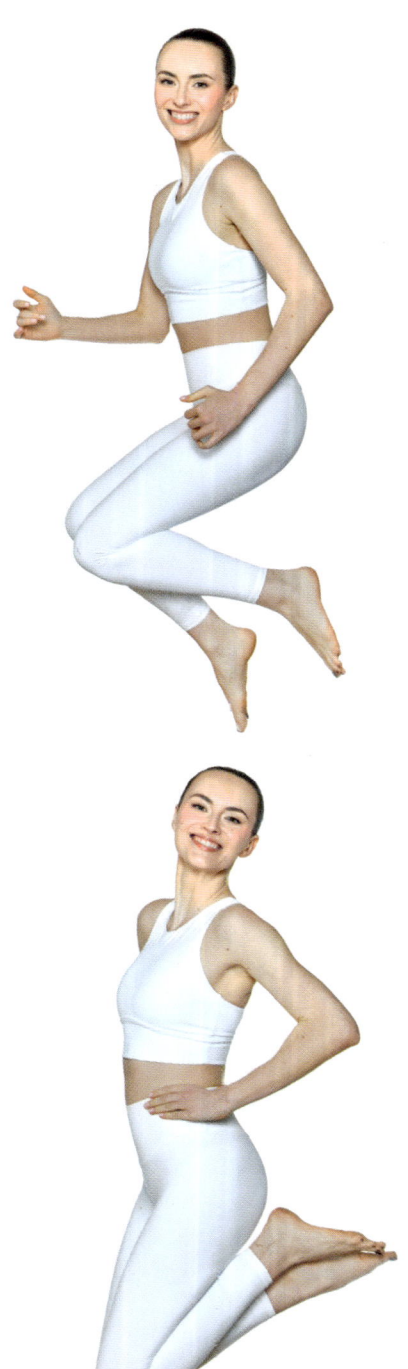

 100 REPS

100 Jumps

Boost your energy & get your lymph moving

This energizing full-body movement activates your lymphatic system, reduces puffiness, and supports natural detox. It's a powerful way to start your day with more vitality and flow.

1 Prepare
Stand tall with your feet hip-width apart. Soften your knees and relax your shoulders and face. Breathe deeply through your nose.

2 Choose your motion
If your knees are healthy, begin with small, springy jumps. If you have any knee issues or joint sensitivity, stomp gently by lifting your heels and pressing them down into the floor with rhythm. If you have a fuller bust, hold your chest gently with your hands to prevent discomfort. Otherwise, keep your arms relaxed by your sides or place your hands where they feel most natural.

3 Bounce and breathe
Begin jumping or stomping. Focus on light, rhythmic motions and steady nasal breathing. Let your entire body join the movement. It's about vibration, not height. Continue for 100 repetitions or until you feel your body has warmed up and awakened.

1 MIN

The Neck Tap

Stimulate your neck's natural flow

This exercise stretches your neck, improves neck wrinkles and jowels, and prevents a double chin. Keeping your neck straight during this exercise will improve the appearance of your neck.

1 Tilt
Tilt – but don't rotate – your head to one side as far as you can, keeping your body straight. Gently look up.

2 Tap
Gently tap from the top of your neck down your neckline towards your shoulders. Keep the tapping light and rhythmic, relax your jaw, and let your breath flow freely throughout.

3 Continue and repeat
Continue this motion for 30 seconds, before switching and repeating on the other side for a further 30 seconds. Keep breathing, relax your shoulders, and enjoy the sensation.

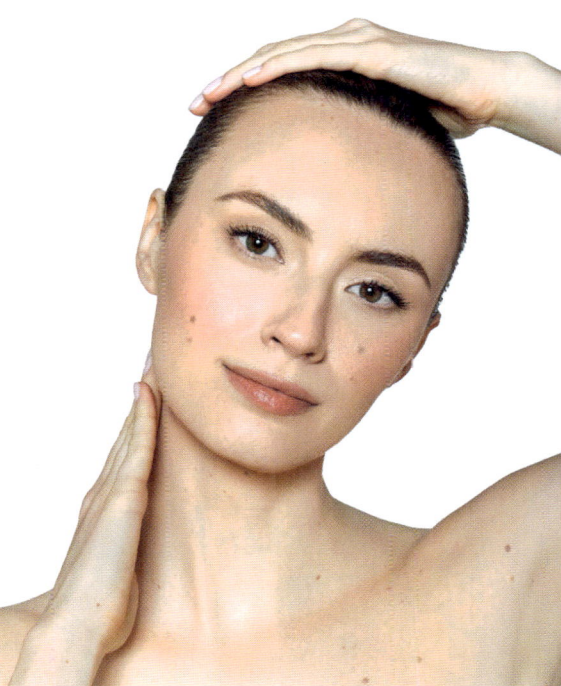
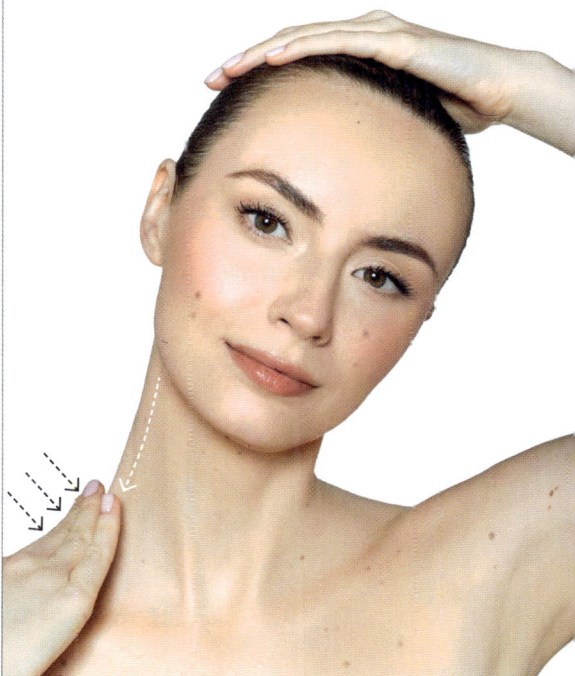

THE METHOD & MOVEMENTS

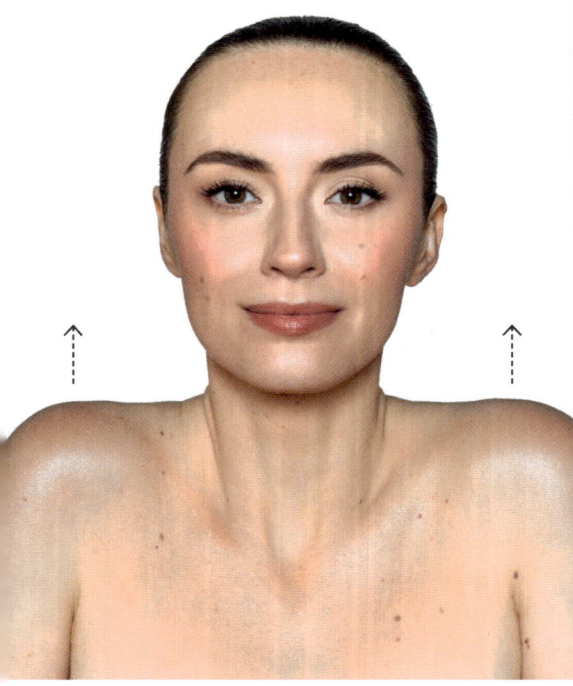
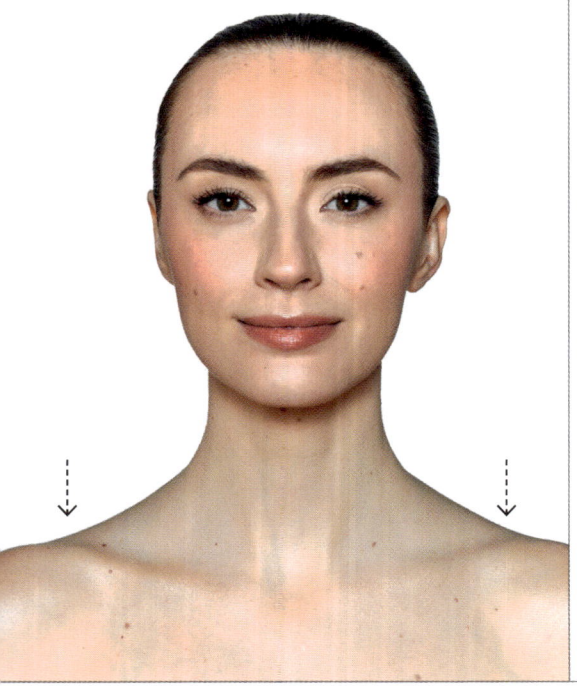

 1 MIN

The Shoulder Warm-Up

Wake up the shoulders & boost circulation

This is an excellent way to release built-up tension from stress or poor posture, support proper lymphatic drainage, and prepare your upper body for deeper face and posture work.

1 Lift your shoulders
Pull your shoulders up towards your ears, pause for a second, then drop the shoulders back down. Make sure you lift both shoulders evenly, and to the same height.

2 Repeat
Continue at your own pace for 1 minute, keeping your neck and face relaxed, and your breathing slow and steady.

> **TIP**
> *As you drop your shoulders down, exhale with intention. Imagine releasing any stress you've been holding there.*

FACE YOGA

1 MIN

The Neck Warm-Up

Gently release tension from your neck

This warm-up helps unlock neck and jaw stiffness, encourages smoother movement, and brings awareness to posture. It sets the stage for deeper facial exercises by loosening your body up.

1 Move to one side
Slowly turn your head to one side as far as is comfortably possible.

2 Move to the other side
Gently turn your head to the other side, reaching your maximum range without strain.

3 Repeat
Continue this smooth left-to-right movement at a calm, steady pace for 1 minute. Don't forget to breathe, and relax your jaw.

> **TIP**
> Keep your jaw soft and lips slightly parted throughout. This helps prevent clenching and allows for a more natural range of motion.

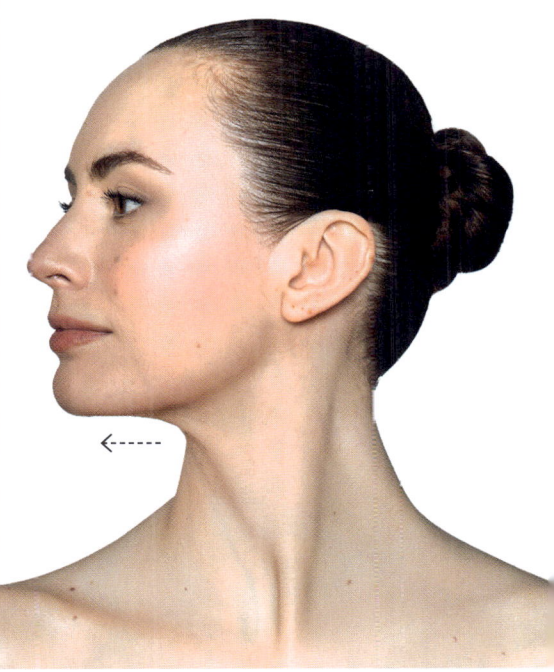

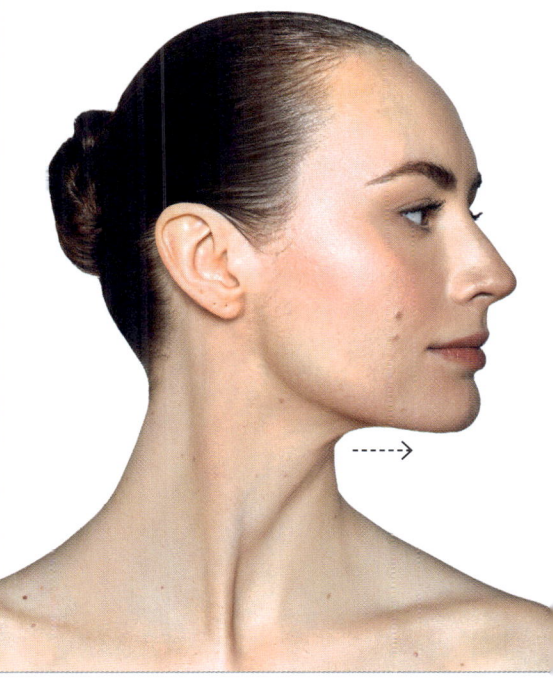

THE METHOD & MOVEMENTS

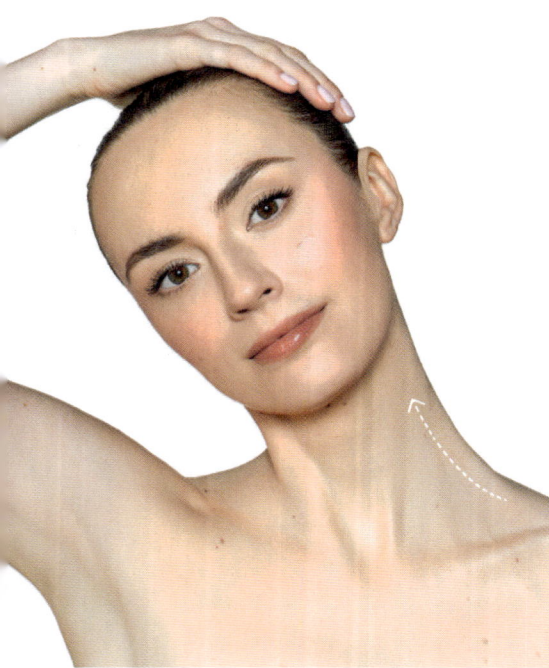

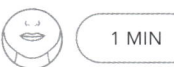 1 MIN

The Neck Stretch

Unwind upper body tightness

This exercise releases tension in the neck and shoulders. Elongating these muscles supports better posture, increases circulation to the face, and relieves the pressure that can contribute to jaw tension and facial asymmetry.

1 Tilt your head
Tilt (but don't rotate) your head to one side as far as you can, imagining that you are trying to touch your shoulder with your ear. Gently place your hand on the top side of your head. Feel the stretch and breathe into it, holding this position for 30 seconds.

2 Switch sides
Repeat on the other side for 30 seconds. Don't forget to breathe, and do not tuck your chin in. Ease into the pose, and enjoy the sensation.

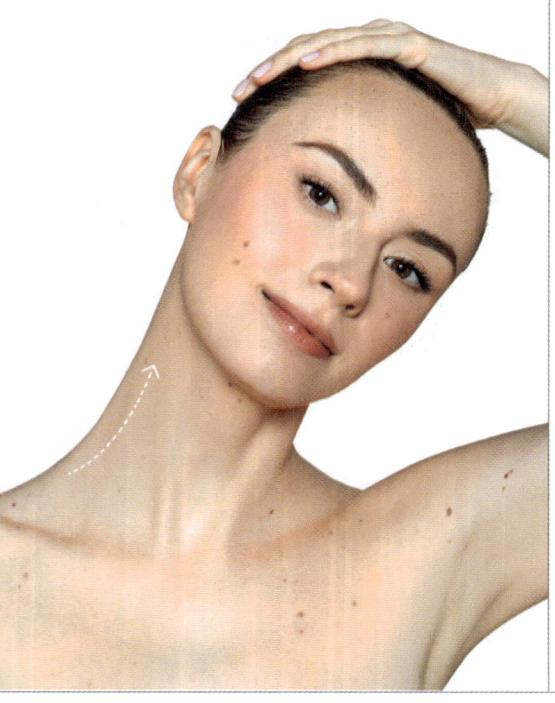

1 MIN

The Knuckle Rotation

Loosen neck tension & restore mobility

This exercise can relax your neck, warm it up, and stimulate blood flow. It helps release muscular tension, support lymphatic flow, and improve mobility in areas that often hold stress.

1 Place your fists
Make a loose fist with both hands and place them along the back and sides of your neck.

2 Rotate
Gently rotate your hands to massage your neck. Glide your knuckles evenly up and down your neck while rotating them at your own pace. This should feel nice and release tension. You can tilt your head from one side to another or look up and down.

3 Massage
Continue for 1 minute, analysing where you are holding tension and focusing on those points. Don't forget to breathe, and keep your chest open.

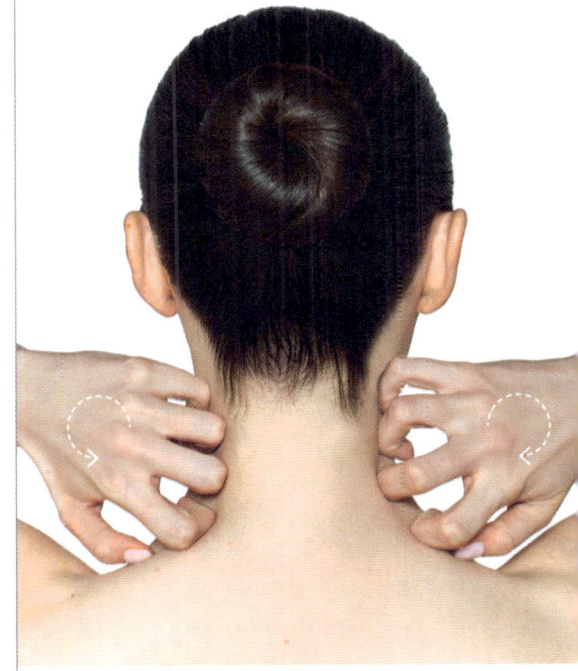

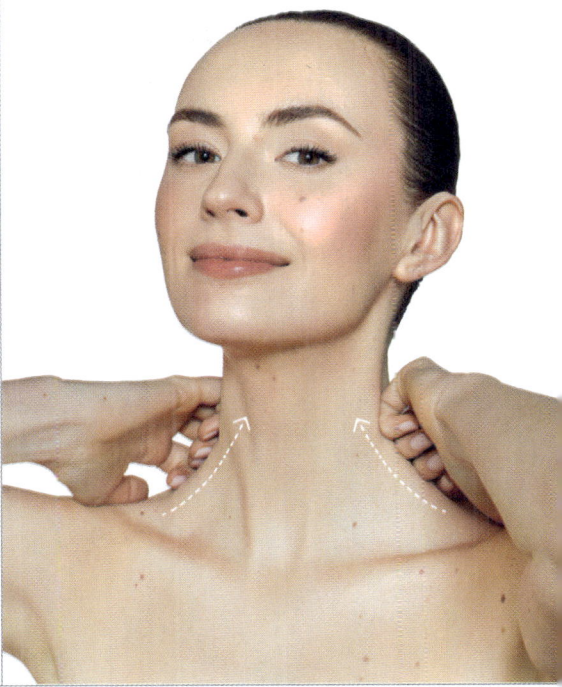

THE METHOD & MOVEMENTS

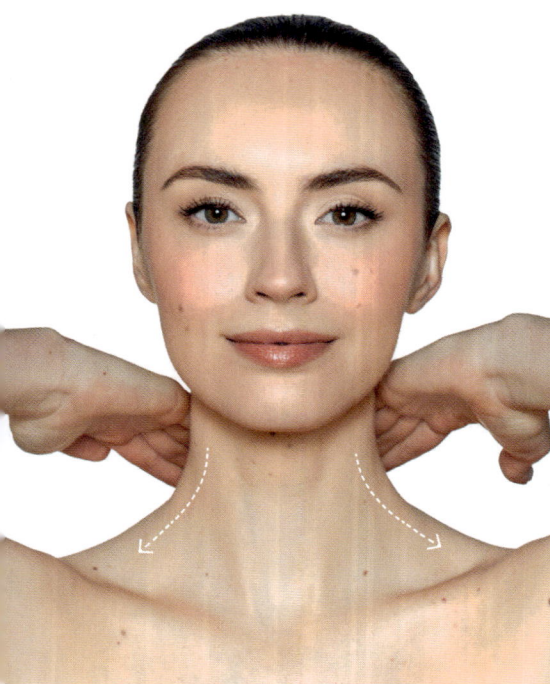
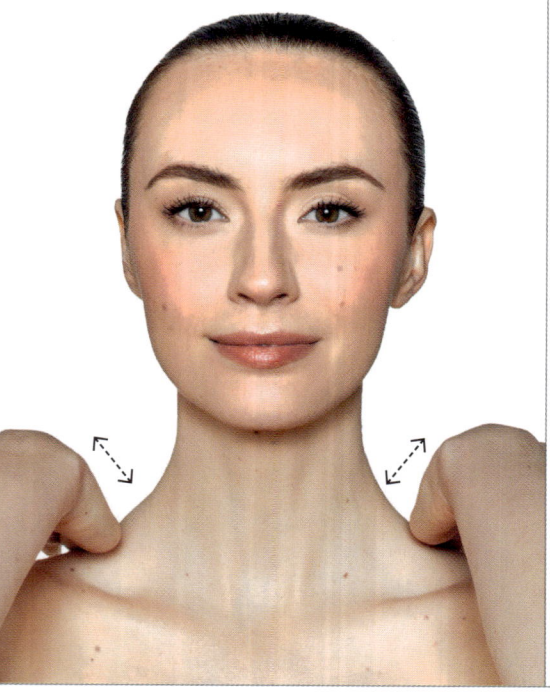

 1 MIN

The Ballerina Neck

Achieve a more lifted, radiant appearance

The neck is extremely important for the look of our faces, and if it becomes tense, it will inhibit blood circulation and lymphatic drainage, which, after a while, will show on your face. This exercise gently helps get the blood and lymph moving.

1 Place your hands
Flatten your hands, and place the outer edges (next to your pinky finger) at the back and sides of your neck, so that your fingers rest towards the nape of your neck.

2 Massage
Keeping your hands flat, move the hands back and forwards to massage the muscles with the outer edges of your hand, going up and down the neck, and stopping at the upper shoulder. Don't massage your spine, but the muscles right next to it.

3 Find your rhythm
You can tilt your head up or down while doing this exercise. Enjoy the sensation, focus on releasing tension in your neck, and adjust the pressure to suit you. Continue for 1 minute.

1 MIN

The Heart Opener Stretch

Improve posture & boost energy in your face

This simple yet powerful posture reset opens your chest, counters the effects of hunching, and boosts circulation to the face. It's a great move to do anytime you feel tense, closed, or low-energy.

1 Position your arms
Interlace your fingers behind your back so your palms face each other. If this is too intense, you can hold a towel or strap between your hands instead.

2 Open your chest
Straighten your arms and slowly lift your hands away from your back. As you do, gently pull your shoulder blades together and feel your chest expand.

3 Lift and lengthen
Keep your chin slightly lifted and your gaze straight ahead or upwards. Breathe deeply through your nose and feel the stretch across your chest and the front of your shoulders. Avoid arching your lower back. Keep your spine long and neutral. Stay in this position for 1 minute continuing to breathe deeply. When you're ready, slowly release your arms and roll your shoulders.

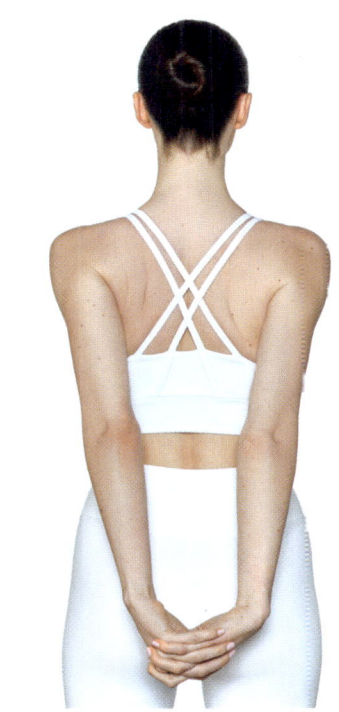

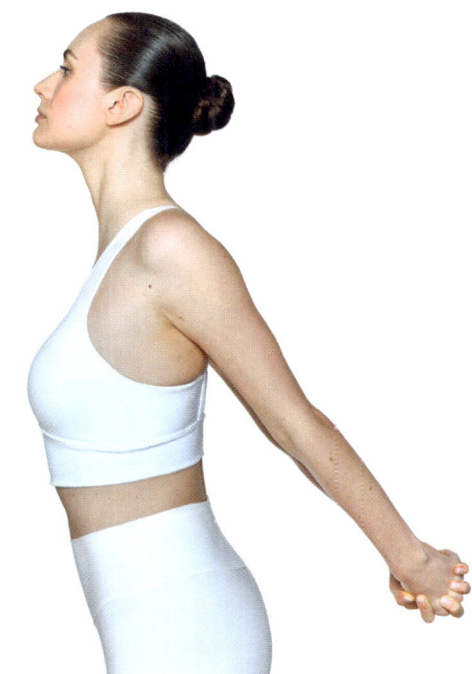

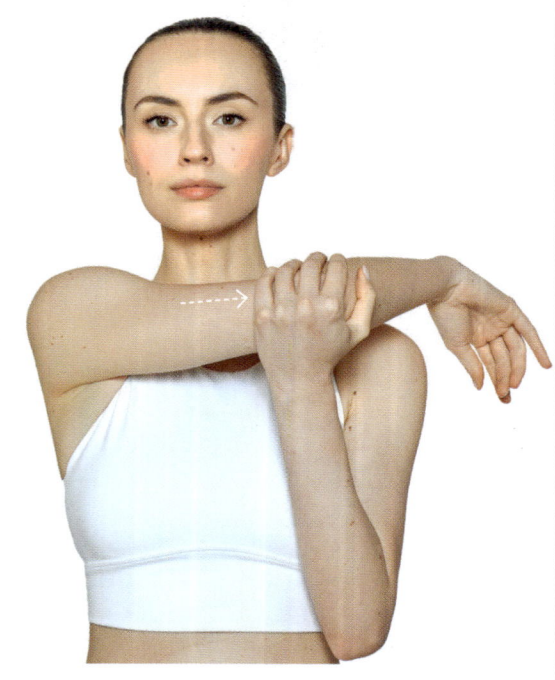

 1 MIN

The Shoulder Hug Stretch

Soften shoulder stiffness & ease your posture

This simple stretch releases built-up tension in the back of the shoulders, improves flexibility, and helps relax upper-body tightness caused by long hours of sitting or screen time.

1 **Lift and stretch**
Raise your right arm out in front of you, and then use your left hand to gently pull your right elbow across your chest towards your left shoulder. Keep your neck relaxed and spine upright, and allow your right hand to relax down.

2 **Breathe and hold**
Hold this stretch for 30 seconds, feeling a gentle pull in the back of your right shoulder. Continue breathing deeply and keep your face soft.

3 **Switch sides**
Release slowly and repeat on the other side for another 30 seconds.

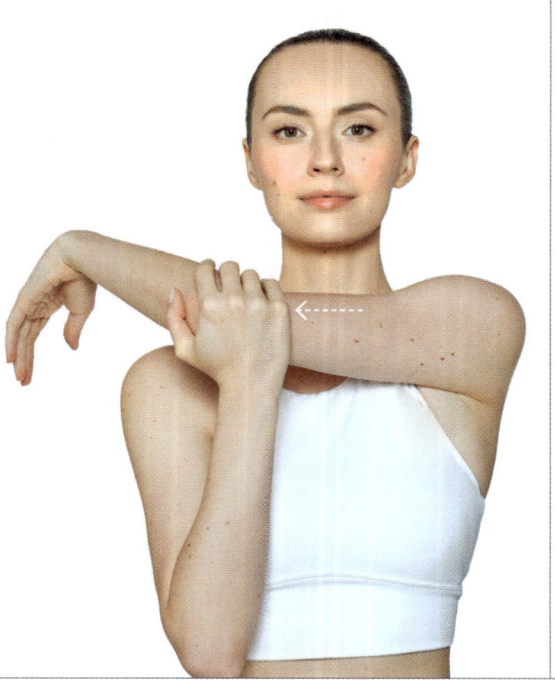

1 MIN

The Diagonal Neck Release

Ease neck & built-up tension

This gentle stretch targets deep neck stiffness and enhances flexibility. It's perfect for unwinding tight muscles, especially if you've been holding stress in your shoulders or working at a screen.

1 Turn and tilt
Gently look diagonally down towards the right side, as if you're glancing towards your hip or underarm.

2 Place your hand
Place your right hand gently onto the back of your head.

3 Stretch and breathe
Apply light pressure with your hand to deepen the stretch. You should feel it along the back and side of your neck. Breathe deeply and avoid pulling. The sensation should feel like a release, not strain.

4 Hold and switch
Hold the stretch for 30 seconds, then slowly release and repeat on the other side.

> **TIP**
> Try this in the evening or before bed to melt away tension from the day.

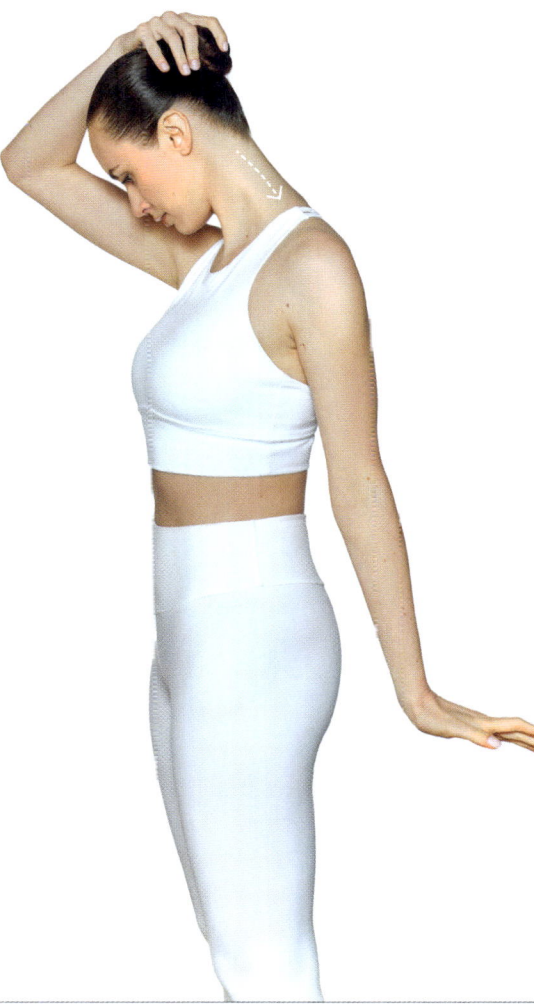

THE METHOD & MOVEMENTS

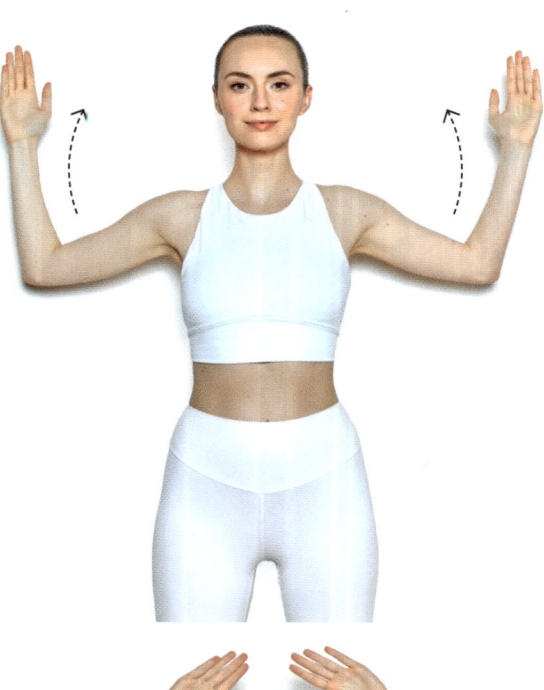
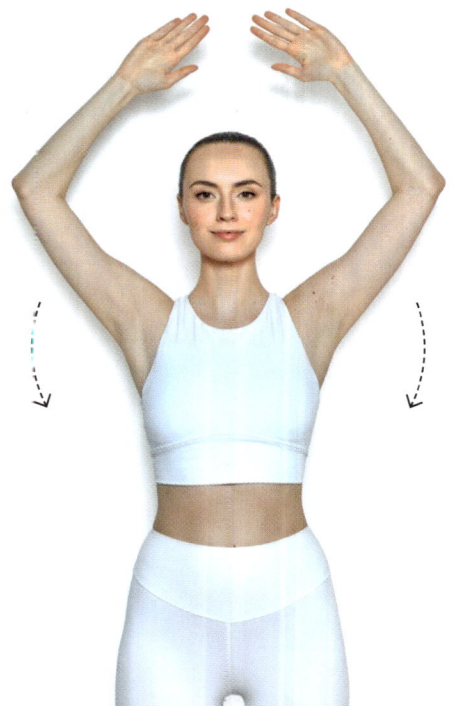

 10-15 REPS

The Angel Wings

Reconnect with your posture

This movement opens your chest, strengthens postural muscles, and glides the fascia of your upper back and arms. It's ideal for anyone who slouches or sits for long hours.

1 Position yourself
Stand with your back flat against a wall, your feet about a foot away from the wall, and your knees slightly bent. Gently tuck your chin and lengthen the back of your neck.

2 Align your arms
Raise both arms to shoulder height and bend your elbows to 90 degrees, creating a goalpost or cactus shape. Press the backs of your hands, elbows, and shoulders into the wall, or as close as your body allows.

3 Make angel wings
Slowly slide your arms upwards towards the sky, and so that your hands almost touch above your head, like angel wings. Keep your elbows and hands in contact with the wall as much as possible. Once your arms are extended as far as you can go without arching your back, slowly glide them back down to the starting position. Repeat the move for 10-15 slow reps, keeping your spine long, ribs gently tucked, and avoiding letting your lower back peel off the wall.

1 MIN

The Armpit & Arm Opener

Create space for breath & flow

This stretch targets the often-overlooked armpit and upper arm area, which are vital zones for mobility, lymph flow, and emotional release. It also boosts circulation through your upper body.

1. **Relax**
   Stand tall with your feet shoulder-width apart. Distribute your weight evenly and soften your knees. Open your chest, breathe deeply, and let your face relax.

2. **Lift your arm**
   Raise your right elbow up towards the ceiling, allowing your hand to fall gently down behind your head.

3. **Stretch and breathe**
   Use your left hand to gently hold the right elbow. Feel the stretch along your upper arm and through your armpit area. Keep your neck soft and shoulders down. Hold this for 30 seconds.

4. **Switch sides**
   Release slowly, then repeat the same movement on the left side for another 30 seconds.

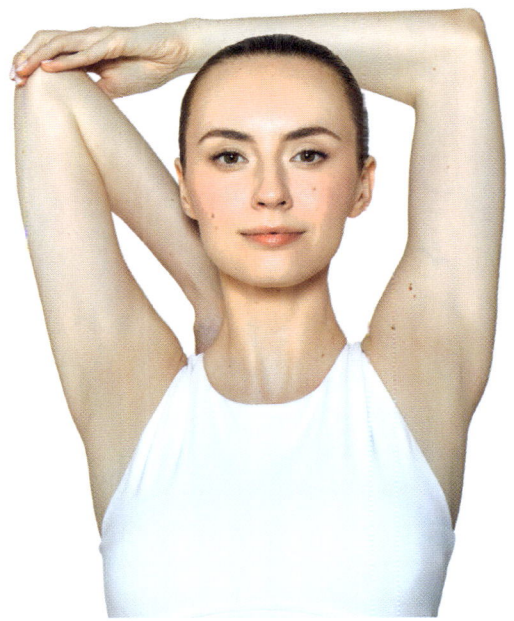

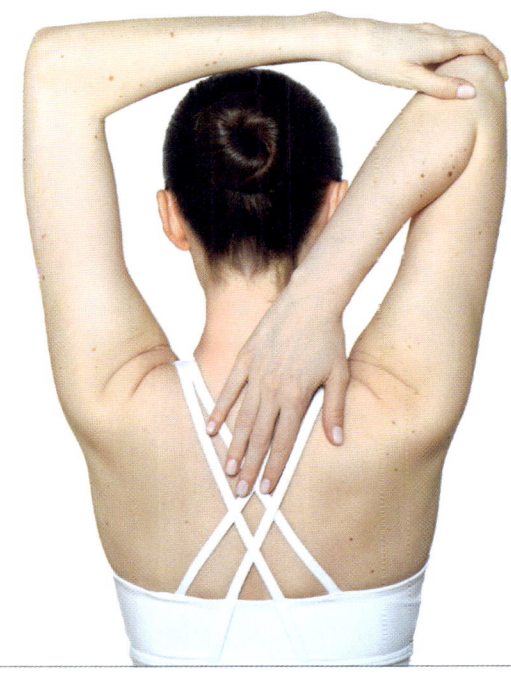

THE METHOD & MOVEMENTS

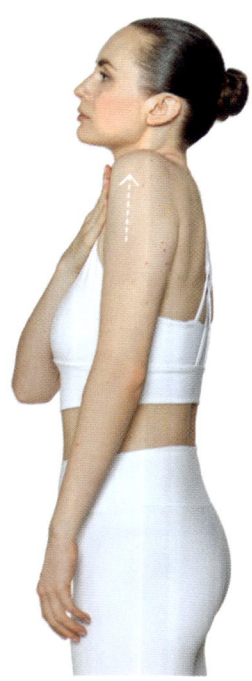
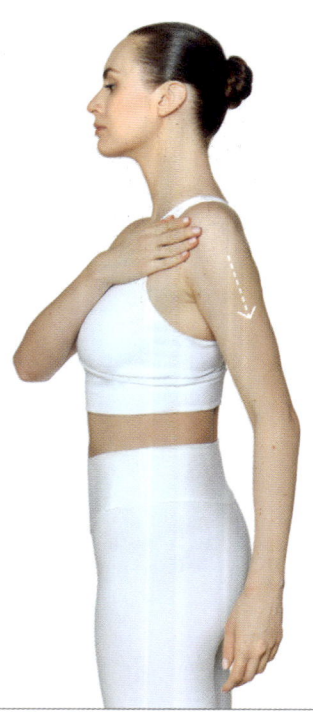

 30-40 REPS

The Shoulder Realigner

Retrain your shoulders for upright posture

This subtle but powerful movement retrains your shoulders for better alignment, and releases built-up tension, perfect for reversing the effects of slouching or habits like carrying a bag on one side.

1 Lift your shoulder
Raise your left shoulder slowly up towards your left ear.

2 Guide the motion
Place your right hand on the front of your raised shoulder and gently guide it back and slightly down as you release it. The right shoulder should stay relaxed. You're not creating resistance, just helping the left shoulder glide into a more aligned position.

3 Repeat
Continue this guided movement, lifting the shoulder up, then gently pressing it back and down with your opposite hand. Breathe steadily as you repeat 15–20 times.

4 Switch sides
Relax and repeat the same sequence on the right side 15–20 times, using your left hand to guide the motion. Focus on fluidity and releasing built-up tension.

1 MIN

The Standing Chest Stretch

TIP

Perfect after long hours at the computer or extended travel, when the body tends to slump forwards.

Open your chest & reset your posture

This stretch opens the front of your chest and shoulders, which are areas that often shorten due to slouching or screen time. It's a powerful posture reset that also encourages deeper breathing.

1 Position yourself
Stand tall next to a wall. Raise your right arm to shoulder height and place your palm and forearm flat against the wall, with your elbow bent at a 90-degree angle.

2 Open your chest
Turn your upper body away from the wall, keeping your spine straight and your shoulder down. Position your feet so that they are parallel to the wall. You should feel a deep stretch through your chest.

3 Hold and breathe
Maintain this position and breathe slowly and deeply through your nose. Keep your body aligned and avoid leaning or twisting too far. The movement shouldn't feel forced.

4 Release and switch
Hold the stretch for 30 seconds, then slowly return to centre and repeat on the other side for 30 seconds

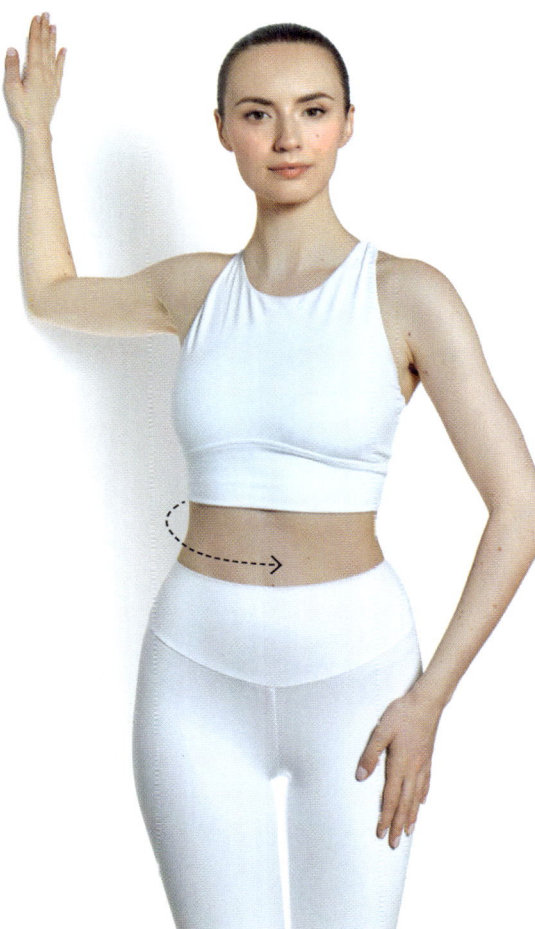

THE METHOD & MOVEMENTS

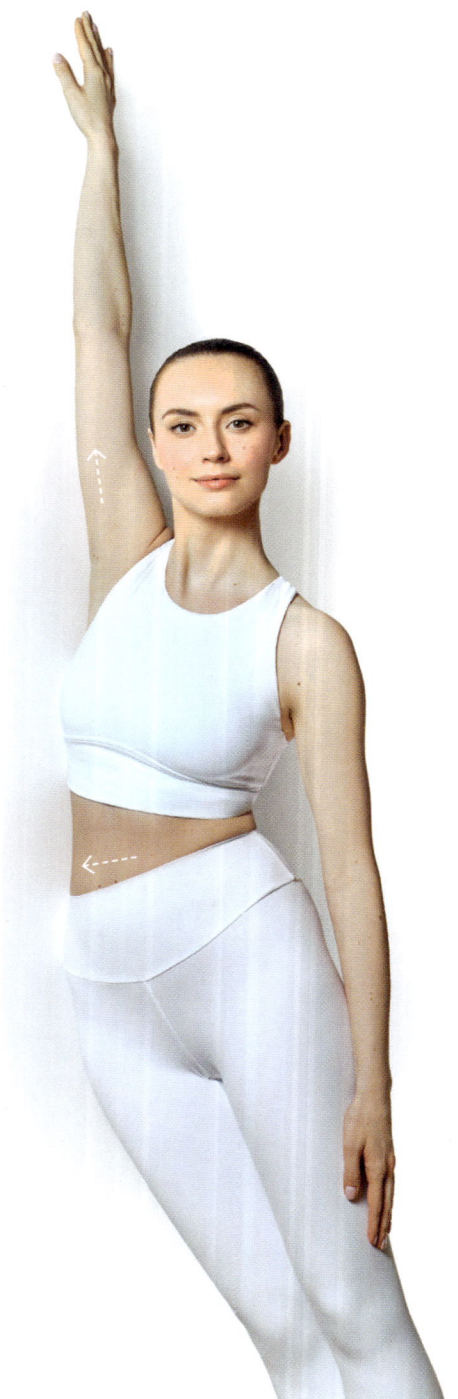

 1 MIN

The Wall Side Stretch

Create space through your entire side body

This stretch opens your armpits, ribs, and waist, which are areas often compressed from poor posture or shallow breathing. It improves flexibility and promotes a sense of upper-body length.

1 Position yourself
Stand sideways next to a wall with your feet hip-width apart and firmly grounded. Keep your hips squared forwards.

2 Lift and reach
Raise the arm closest to the wall and stretch it upwards, bringing your bicep close to your ear. Extend your arm towards the ceiling, and place the side of your body lightly against the wall for support.

3 Lean into the stretch
Press your armpit and side ribs into the wall and begin to lean slightly into it, creating a stretch along the entire side of your body.

4 Breathe and release
Take steady, deep breaths and feel the stretch. Hold for 30 seconds, then gently release, and repeat on the opposite side for 30 seconds.

2 MIN

The Standing Chest Glide

Open your chest & melt shoulder tension

This stretch and fascia gliding technique releases tension from the chest and shoulders. It's ideal for opening the front body, improving posture, and restoring freedom of movement.

1 Position yourself
Stand next to a wall, raise your right arm to shoulder height and place your palm and forearm flat against the wall, with your elbow bent at a 90-degree angle.

2 Open your chest
Gently rotate your chest away from the wall to feel a stretch across your chest and the front of your right shoulder. Position your feet so that they are parallel to the wall.

3 Turn your head
Slowly turn your head to look to the wall, deepening the stretch through your neck.

4 Add the glide
With your left hand, begin a slow glide from the centre of your chest out towards your left shoulder. Continue for 1 minute.

5 Switch sides
Repeat on the other side for 1 minute.

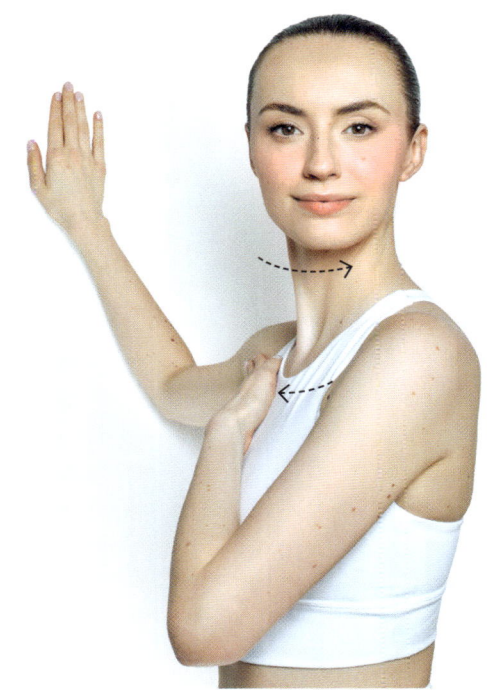

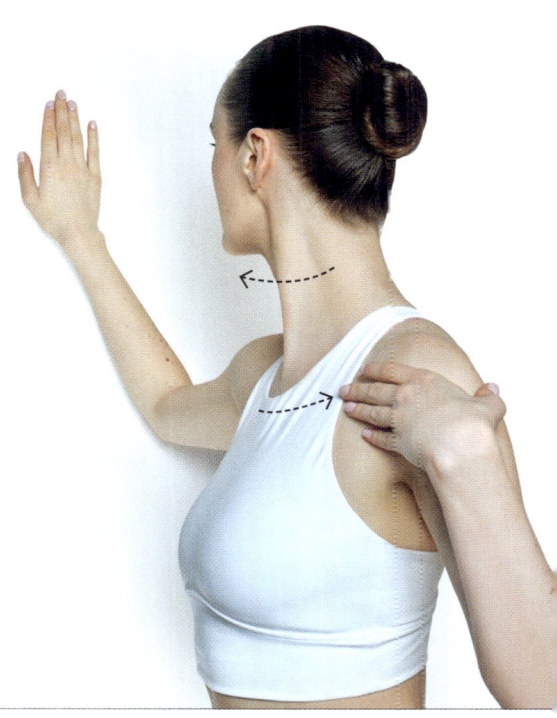

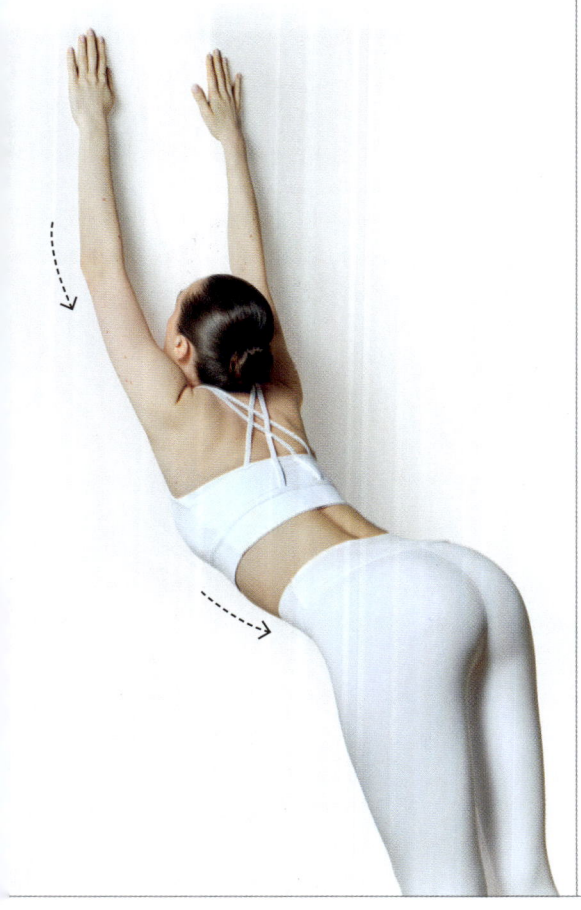

3-4 REPS

Wall Shoulder Chest Opener

Unwind your upper body tension

This stretch releases tightness in the entire upper body. It helps rehydrate fascia, decompress your spine, and open your chest, which is perfect for improving posture and enhancing mobility.

1 Position yourself
Stand facing a wall with your feet hip-width apart and 30–40 cm (12–16 in) away from the wall. Place both arms on the wall high above your head, and shoulder-width apart.

2 Start the glide
Begin gliding your arms down the wall in a controlled motion. Let your back round and your chest open as you fold forwards. As your arms glide downwards, feel the stretch ripple through your chest, upper back, shoulders, and spine.

3 Hold at the bottom
Pause at your lowest comfortable point and take a few steady breaths. Let your body melt deeper into the stretch with each exhale.

4 Return and repeat
Slowly glide your arms back up the wall, restack your spine, and repeat the movement 2–3 more times.

2 MIN

The Neck Reset

Undo deep neck tension & reset your posture

This technique stretches and releases the upper neck and back area. It's especially effective if you're prone to a neck hump, or spend a lot of time at a desk or on your phone.

1 **Activate and breathe**
Stand, look up, and carefully tilt your head back as far as you can. You can hold onto the your waist tissue for support, but keep your shoulders relaxed. Hold the stretch until you feel the tension building up.

2 **Release and reposition**
Release the stretch, look forwards, and place both of your hands on the back right side of the neck, with the left hand on top.

3 **Stretch the tissue**
Tilt your head gently towards the left shoulder, and apply strong pressure to your fingers. Using deep, slow strokes, move the fascia and muscles by gliding the top hand up to the ear, and the bottom hand down to the edge of the shoulder. Apply steady pressure and stretch the tissue, pausing and focusing on any tighter areas.

4 **Breathe and finish**
Repeat this stretch for 1 minute, then repeat on the right side for 1 minute.

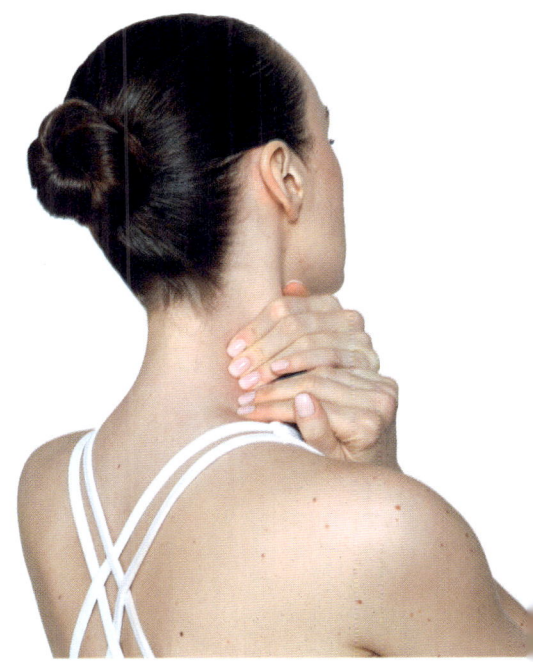

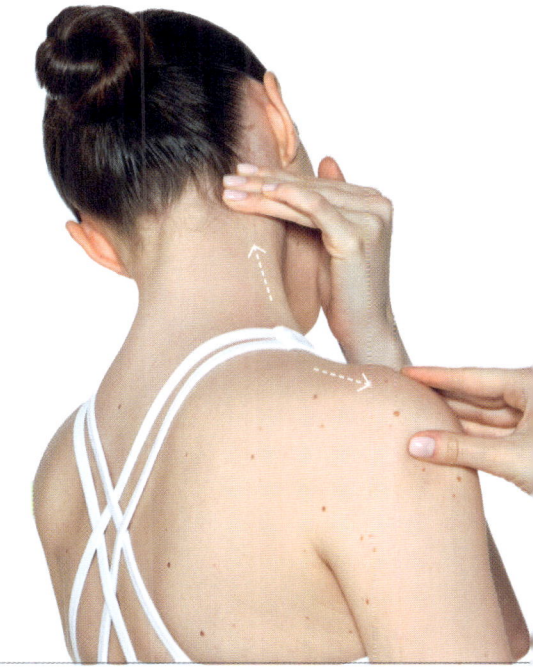

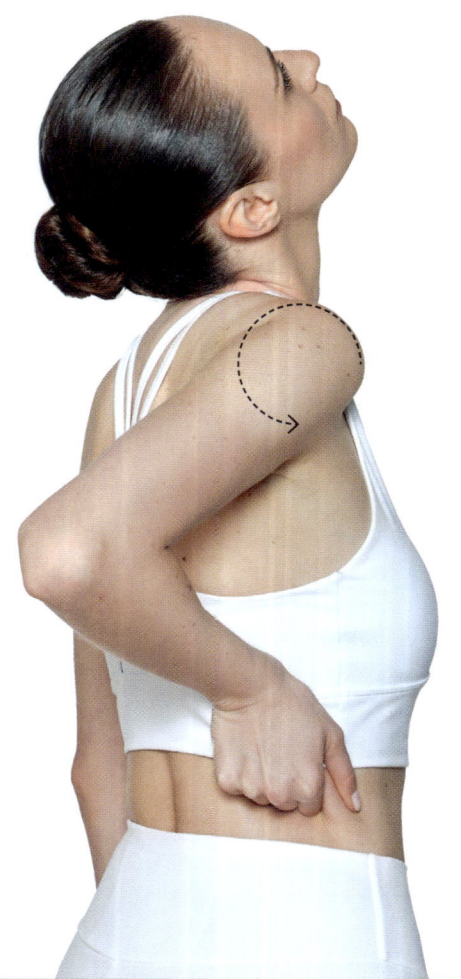

 60-80 REPS

The Shoulder Spiral

Loosen tension & reset your posture

This exercise targets shoulder mobility and fascial release, helping to reduce upper-body stiffness that often contributes to facial tension, jaw clenching, and forward head posture.

1. Place your hand
Place your right hand on your waist or hip and gently look up. Keep your elbow relaxed and pointing slightly out to the side.

2. Start the rotation
Begin rotating your right shoulder in large, slow circles, 15-20 times in one direction. Focus on smooth motion and connection through your shoulder blade and chest.

3. Switch direction
Reverse the rotation and move in the opposite direction for another 15-20 circles. Let the movement feel fluid and tension-free.

4. Switch sides
Repeat on the the left shoulder.

4-6 REPS

The Neck Resistance Press

Improve head alignment & reduce neck strain

This technique strengthens and trains upright posture. The resistance band activates the back line of the body, encouraging better alignment and long-term support for the neck and face.

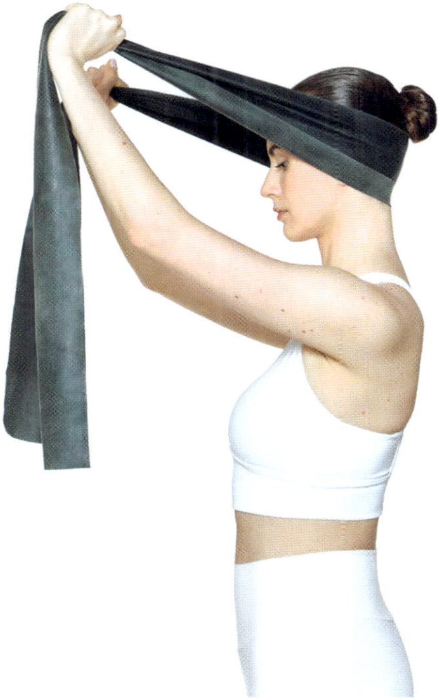

1 Set up your band
Grab a resistance band (like a Terra band or soft pair of leggings). Stand tall and wrap the band around the back of the slightly curved bony area at the base of your skull, just above where your neck begins. Hold the ends of the band out in front of you.

2 Find your posture
Gently tuck your chin and lengthen the back of your neck.

3 Press into resistance
Begin slowly pressing the back of your head into the band, moving your head slightly backwards while keeping your chin slightly down. Imagine drawing your head straight back – not tilting – as you work against the tension of the band.

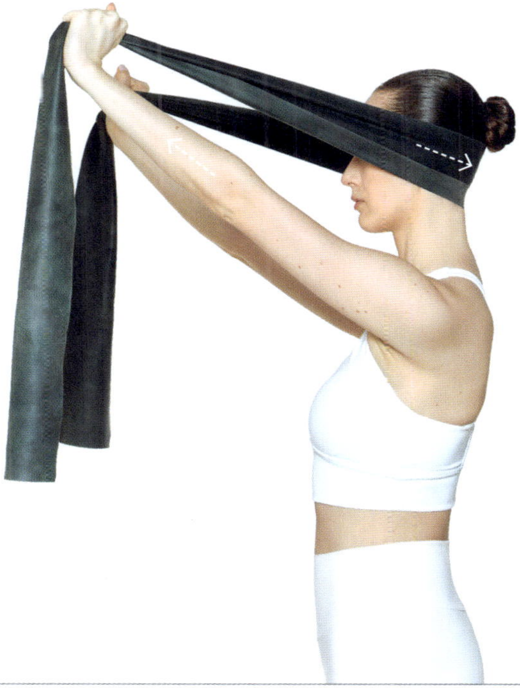

4 Control and breathe
Hold the backwards pressure for 5-8 seconds, then release. Repeat 4-6 times.

PHASE 02
RELEASE TENSION

Your face holds the story of your life in micro-tensions, clenched jaws, furrowed brows, and guarded expressions. These patterns don't just shape how you look – they shape how you feel. In this phase, we'll focus on softening what's been held too tightly for too long.

You'll learn gentle yet powerful techniques to release the layers of tension locked in your fascia and muscles. Like untying a knot, this allows your face to return to its natural position – more open, more balanced, more at ease.

This phase is about clearing the path so that your true expression can shine through.

The SCM Release 76	The Crow's Feet Release 98
The Chest Roll-Ups 77	The Under-Eye Zigzag 99
The Occipital Bone Massage 78	The Hollow Eye Lift 100
The Ear Stretch & Wiggle 79	The Eye Roll Lift 101
The Scalp Shake 80	The Cheek Relaxer 102
The Head Massage 81	The Nasolabial Fold Eraser 103
The Wow 82	The Cheekbone Sculpt 104
The Masseter Relaxer 83	The Cheek Glider 105
The Diagonal Masseter Opener 84	The Cheek Flick 106
The Buccal Massage Release 85	The Cheekbone Definer 107
The Masseter Rolls 86	The Midi Cheek Sculpter 108
The Forehead Tap 87	The Mouth Relaxer 109
The Forehead Massage 88	The Pouty Lip 110
The Forehead Knuckle Glider 89	The Lip Liner 111
The Forehead Glider 90	The Droopy Mouth Release 112
The Frowning X 91	The Chin Smoother 113
The 11 Line Eraser 92	The Mouth & Jaw Tap 114
The Brow Lift Glide 93	The Jawline Hook 115
The Eye Massage 94	The Neck Pinch 116
The Upper Eyelid Depuffer 95	The Midi Jaw Sculpter 117
The Eye Knuckle Glider 96	The Mini Facelift 118
The Eye Depuffer 97	The Happy Cool Down 119

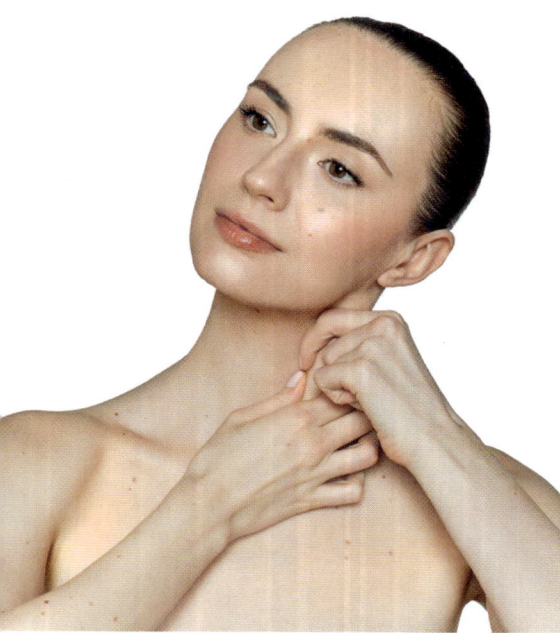

 2 MIN

The SCM Release

Soften neck tension & restore mobility

The sternocleidomastoid (SCM) plays a major role in head and neck movement, and when tight, can cause jaw tension, headaches, and neck stiffness. This massage helps lengthen and release the SCM.

1 **Find the muscle**
Tilt your head slightly to the left, then tilt your chin slightly upwards to the right. A prominent rope-like muscle will pop out at the left side of your neck. That's your SCM.

2 **Grab and stretch**
Hold the muscle between your index fingers and thumbs, so that the left hand is holding towards the centre of the muscle, and the right hand is holding just below.

3 **Glide and release**
With light to medium pressure, slowly glide your left hand up to your ear, and your right hand down the muscle down to your collarbone. Move your hands together for one minute, using a pinching, kneading, or sliding motion. On tender spots, hold gentle pressure for a few seconds.

4 **Repeat and switch sides**
Repeat on the other side for a minute.

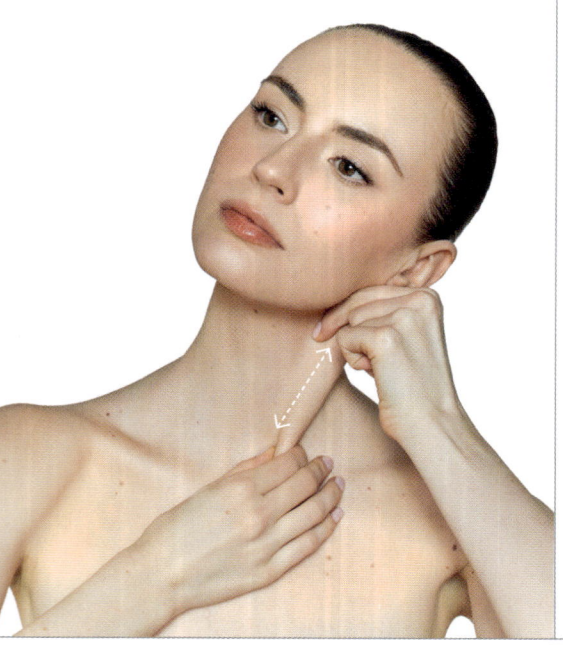

2 MIN

The Chest Roll-Ups

Open the front body & dissolve stored tension

This fascia release technique targets the tissue in your upper chest, which is an area that holds emotional tension and is often compressed by poor posture.

1   **Grab the tissue**
Using your thumbs and index fingers, gently grab the fascia at the centre of your chest, just above the breasts — not just the skin, but the layer beneath. Your thumbs can help anchor as your fingers scoop and lift the tissue.

2   **Roll up**
Without losing contact with the skin, begin to roll the tissue slowly up towards your collarbones. Imagine your fingers creating a continuous wave, lifting, folding, and rolling the fascia upwards like a scroll. Keep your hands in contact with the skin to maintain flow and connection. If the tissue feels stuck or resistant, pause and hold, applying gentle pressure before continuing. Let your breath stay steady and calm as you work.

3   **Repeat**
Continue the rolling motion for 2 minutes, moving across the chest to the other side to cover a different section each time.

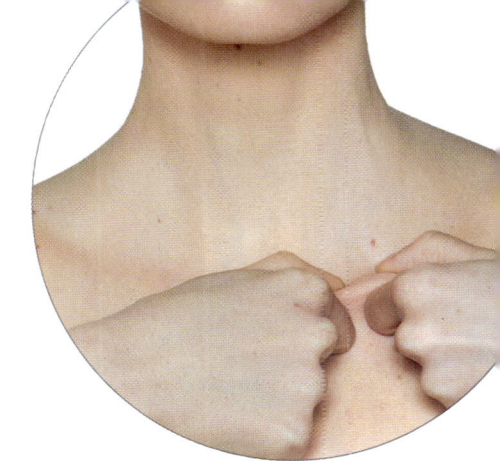
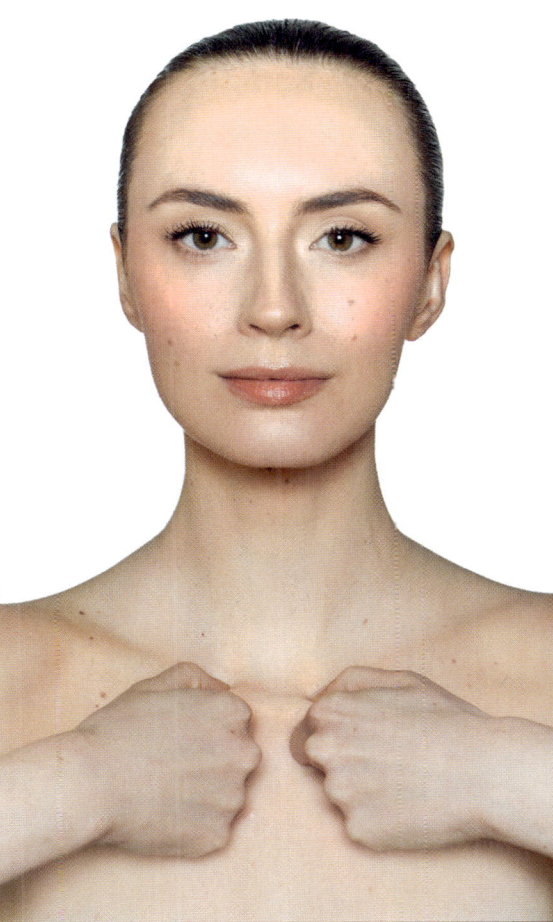

THE METHOD & MOVEMENTS

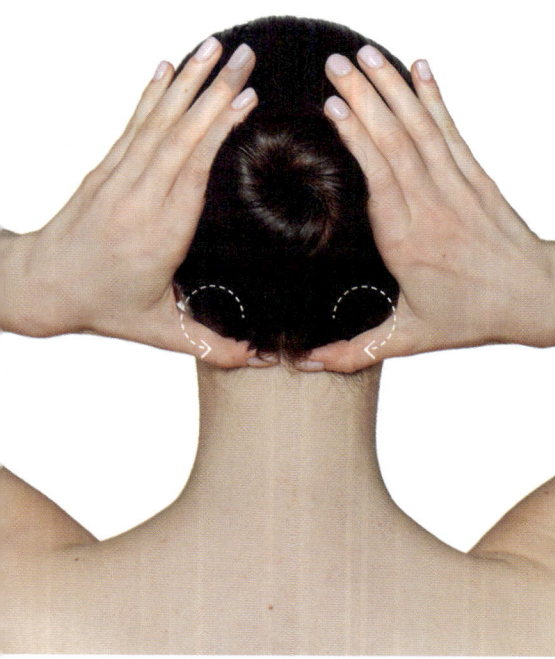
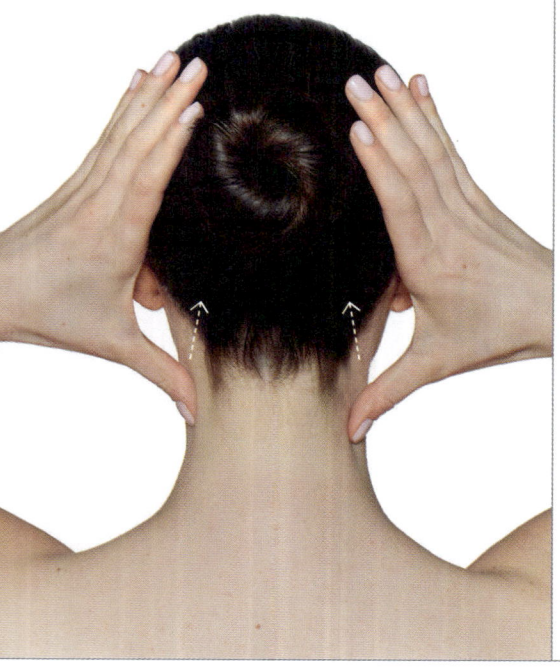

 2 MIN

The Occipital Bone Massage

Release tightness that can cause headaches

This massage targets the base of your skull, where tension from stress, poor posture, or eye strain often accumulates. Releasing the tissue here can help your face feel more lifted and open.

1 Relax and position
Sit or lie down comfortably. Place the pads of your thumbs at the base of your skull, just above your neck. Rest your fingers on the crown of your head.

2 Sink and feel
Using your thumbs, sink gently into the tissue just below the occipital bone.

3 Massage and release
Make small, slow circles with your thumbs, moving along the ridge of the occipital bone from the centre out towards your ears. Use enough pressure to reach the deeper tissue, but not so much that it creates tension. Continue for 1 minute.

4 Stretch and glide
Once the area softens, use your thumbs to glide the tissue up towards the occipital bone, as if lifting it. Repeat across the width of the occipital bone for 1 minute.

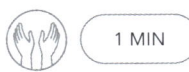 1 MIN

The Ear Stretch & Wiggle

Reset your face, scalp, & nervous system

Your ears are rich in fascia and acupressure points. Stretching and wiggling them can help to release facial tension, improve circulation, and calm the nervous system.

1 Grasp your ears
Gently hold the outer edge of the right ear with your right hand. You can place your other hand on your face for light resistance.

2 Stretch and lengthen
Begin to pull gently but firmly – upwards, outwards, or slightly back – creating a stretch that you feel through the ear and into the scalp and temples. Try changing the angle and direction slowly to explore where you feel the deepest release.

3 Add a wiggle
While maintaining the stretch, add a small circular or side-to-side wiggling motion with your fingers. Keep your touch steady but light.

4 Continue and switch
Continue for about 30 seconds, then switch sides and repeat. You can also finish by gently massaging or tugging on the earlobes to relax the whole system.

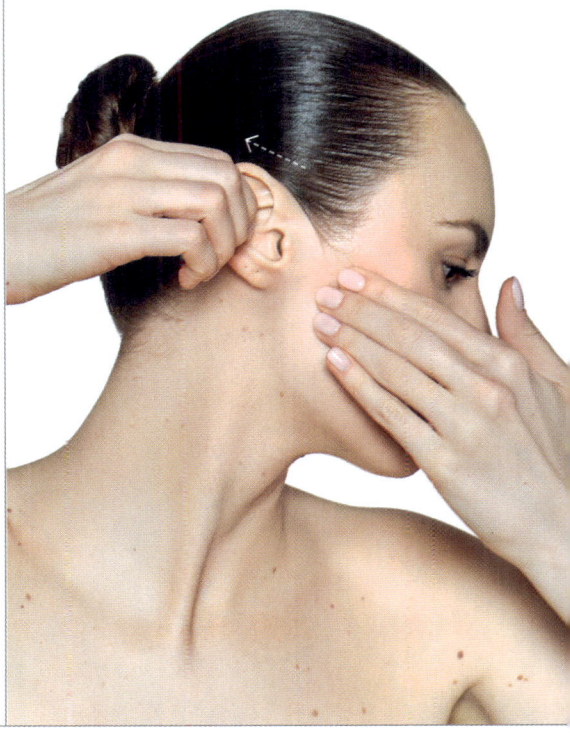

THE METHOD & MOVEMENTS

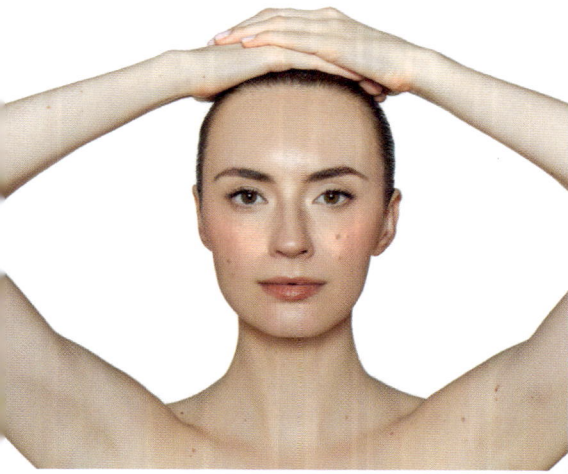
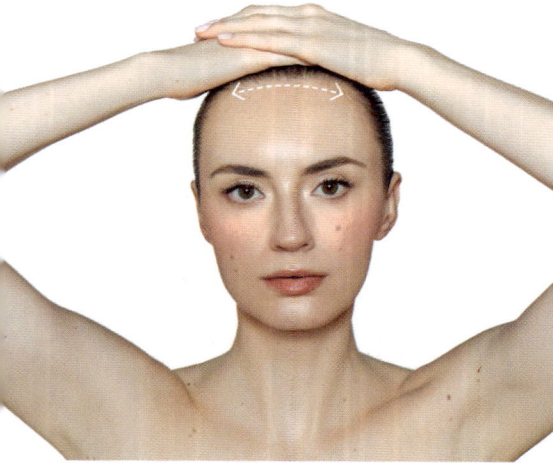
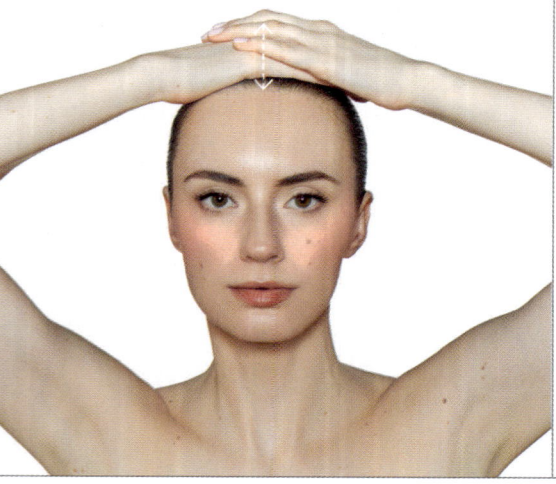

 1 MIN

The Scalp Shake

Stimulate scalp circulation & flexibility

This exercise keeps the skin on your scalp elastic and improves blood circulation, which can also be also beneficial for hair growth.

1   **Place your hands**
Place one hand on top of the other, and rest your bottom palm on top of your head, just beyond your hairline.

2   **Shake from side to side**
Apply pressure into the scalp and move your hands from side to side – creating a gliding motion in the scalp tissue beneath your fingers (not the entire head). Continue for about 20 seconds.

3   **Shake front to back**
Without changing your hand position, start moving the scalp front to back in the same way. Stay grounded, and let the tissue shift beneath your fingertips. Continue for another 20 seconds.

4   **Repeat and finish**
Repeat in either direction (side to side, or forward to back) again for the final 20 seconds, and shift your hands to a new scalp area for more coverage, working your way over the entire scalp.

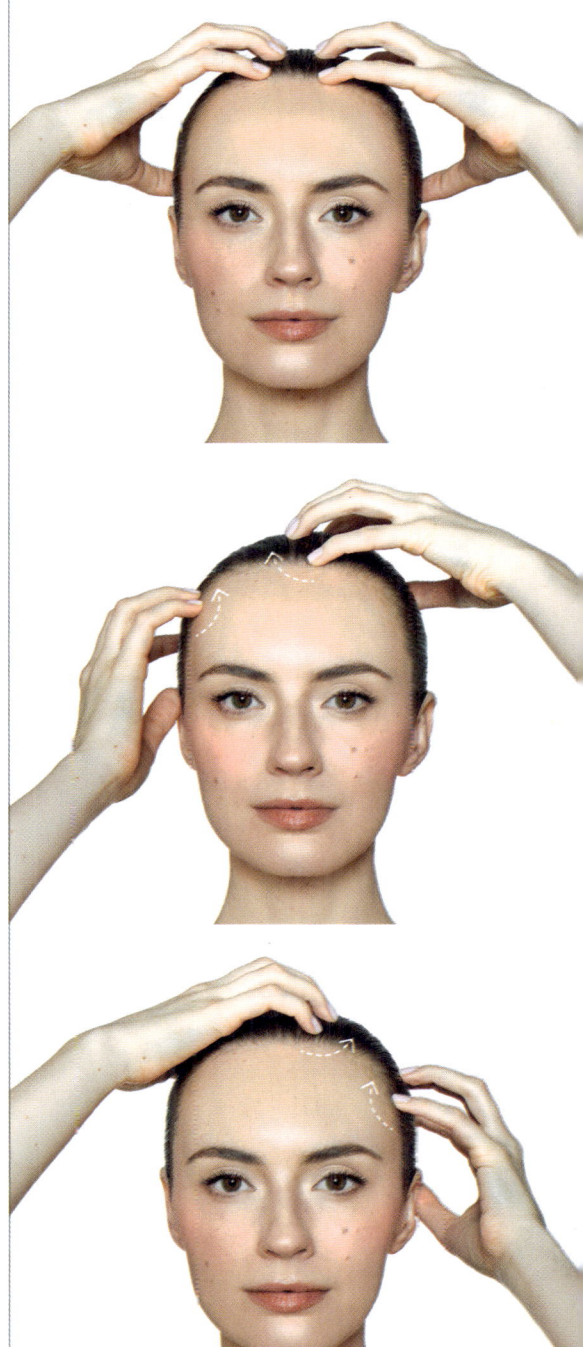

1 MIN

The Head Massage

Wake up your scalp & release deep tension

This exercise improves blood circulation, keeps the skin of the scalp elastic, and improves oxygen flow to the massaged areas.

1 Place your fingertips
Raise both elbows to the side, and place your fingertips onto your scalp, as if you were about to shampoo your scalp.

2 Massage
Using your fingertips, not your nails, apply firm pressure and massage your scalp in circular motions. Massage for 1 minute, starting from the top of your scalp, and moving to the side of your head, then down and across to the back of your scalp.

> **TIP**
> Try to move the skin of your scalp. Don't just rub across the surface. You want to feel the scalp gliding gently over the skull, as that's how you release fascial tension and boost circulation.

THE METHOD & MOVEMENTS

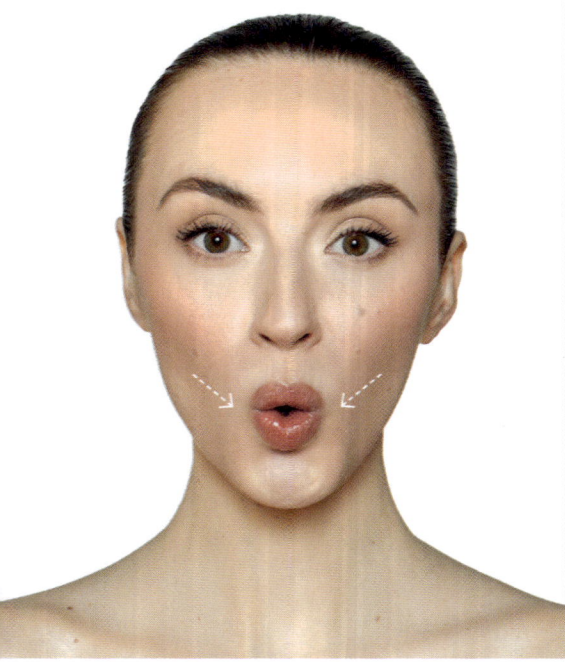

 1 MIN

The Wow

Wake up & energize your whole face

This exercise warms up all facial muscles at once, improving articulation, and boosting your mood. It also helps release tension in the jaw, cheeks, and around the eyes.

1 **Say "Wow"**
Say "Wow" as slowly as you can, and exaggerate the mouth movement as much as possible, opening your eyes as wide as you can without frowning. You should begin with your mouth in a small "o" shape, with the size of the "o" growing to as big as you can stretch it to as you say "Wow".

2 **Repeat**
Continue to repeat "Wow" slowly for one minute. Don't tilt your head, and keep your body still and shoulders relaxed.

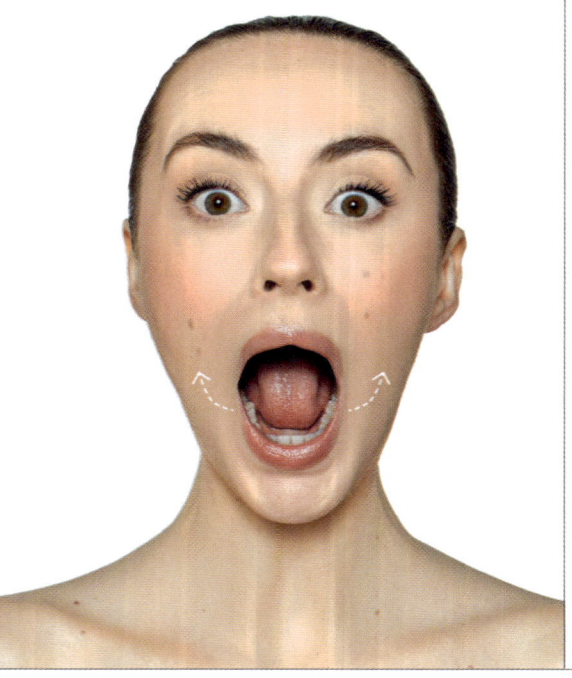

> **TIP**
> *If you notice forehead lines appearing, slow down the movement and soften your effort – less force, more presence.*

1 MIN

The Masseter Relaxer

Release facial puffiness & jaw tightness

The masseter is one of the strongest muscles in your body, and one of the most overused. This deep glide helps soften and reset the masseter, allowing your jaw – and your entire face – to relax.

1 Place your fingers
Place your thumbs underneath either side of your jawbone, and place the inside of the knuckles on your index finger just in front of your ears, on the thick muscle you feel when you clench your jaw. That's your masseter.

2 Glide and open
With your mouth slightly open to help relax the jaw, glide your index knuckles slowly downwards along the masseter towards your jawline. This allows the muscle to lengthen as you work.

3 Repeat
Repeat the motion slowly for 1 minute, increasing depth slightly with each pass if it's comfortable.

> **TIP**
> If one side feels tighter than the other, that's normal. Consistent practice will help bring more balance to your jawline over time.

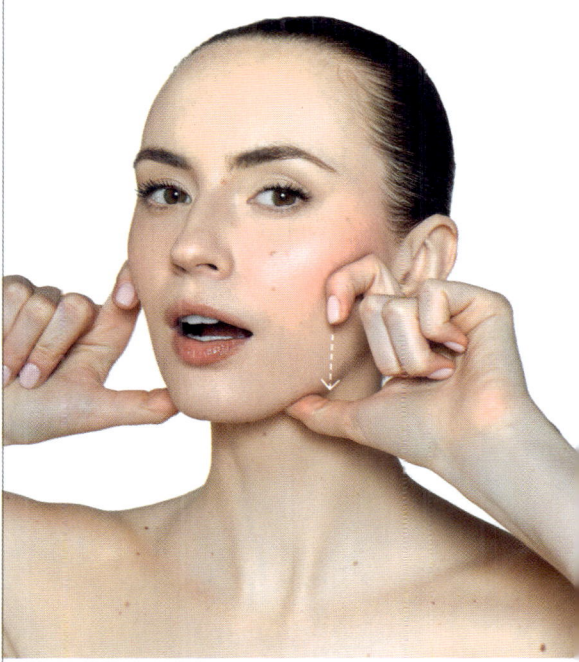
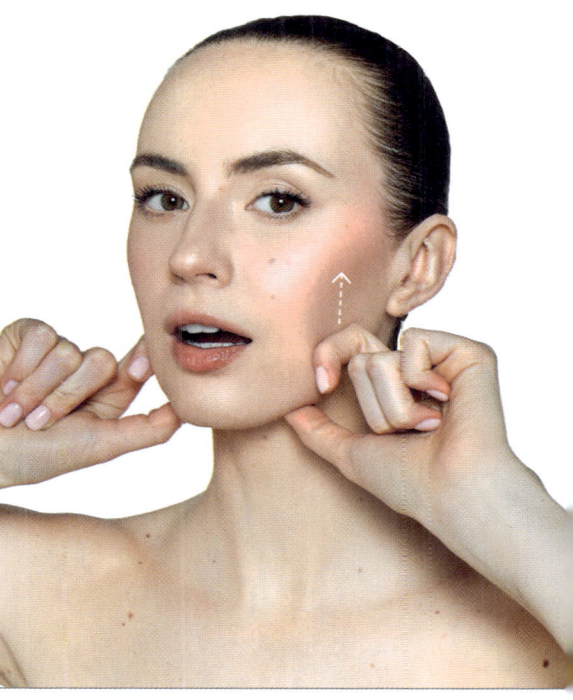

THE METHOD & MOVEMENTS

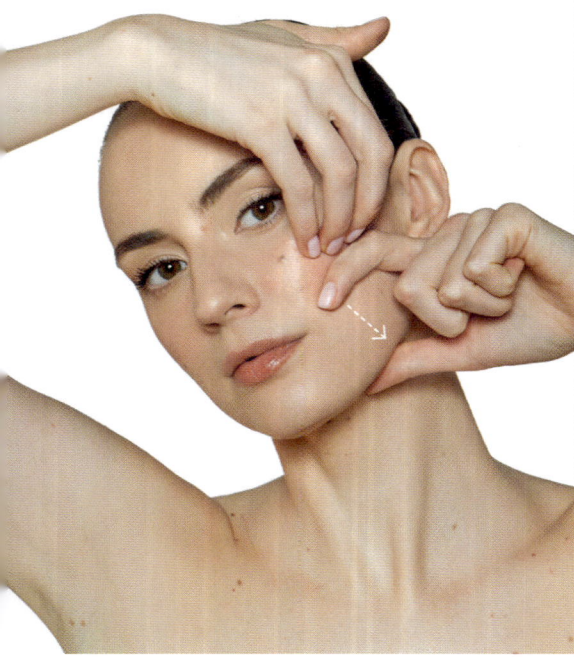
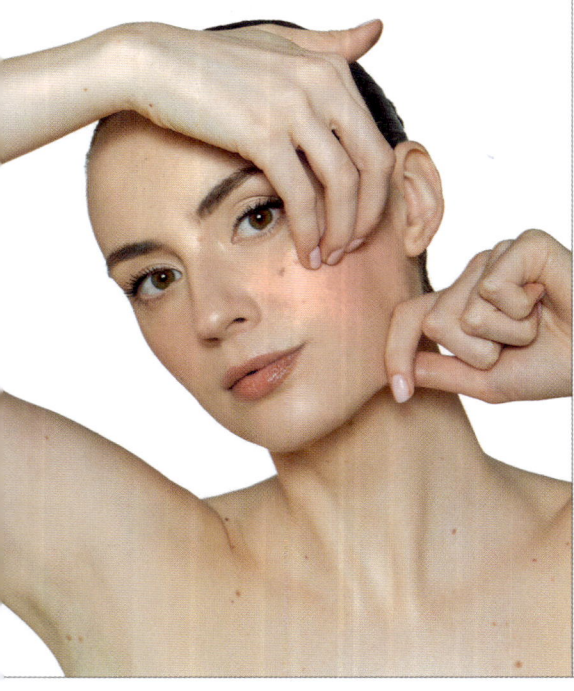

 2 MIN

The Diagonal Masseter Opener

Release deep jaw tension

This masseter release works from your cheek down to your jawline to unlock deep facial tension, encourage healthy circulation, and restore and lift flow in the lower face.

1 Place your fingers
Rest your right forearm across the front of your scalp, until you can place your left ring, middle, and index fingertips on the top of your left cheekbone. Place your left index finger horizontally beneath the right fingertips, where the upper masseter begins. Finally, press your left thumb into the centre left side of your jawbone.

2 Tilt and glide
Gently tilt your head towards the right shoulder to increase the stretch and pressure. Holding your cheek with your right fingertips for support, glide your left finger using firm pressure down your masseter muscle towards your thumb.

3 Repeat and switch sides
Repeat for 1 minute, then repeat on the other side for 1 minute.

2 MIN

The Buccal Massage Release

Bring symmetry back to your cheeks

This release works the masseter and surrounding fascia from the inside out, helping to unlock deep jaw tension, soften a bulky lower face, and bring more lift, circulation, and symmetry to the cheeks.

1 Clean your hands
Always begin with freshly washed hands.

2 Position your hands
Place your left thumb inside your mouth against the inner side of your right cheek, just beside the molars. Use the four fingers of the same hand (on the outside of your face) to gently hold the tissue. This is the outer edge of your masseter muscle.

3 Massage and release
Begin slow, circular or kneading motions with your fingers, working against the thumb inside the cheek. Explore different movements – up, down, or even small pulls – to feel where tension is present.

4 Breathe and switch
Continue for 1 minute, then repeat on the other side for 1 minute.

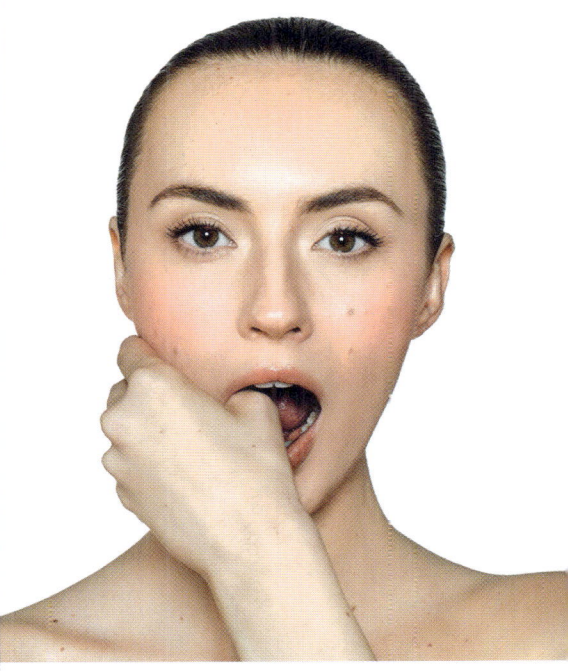
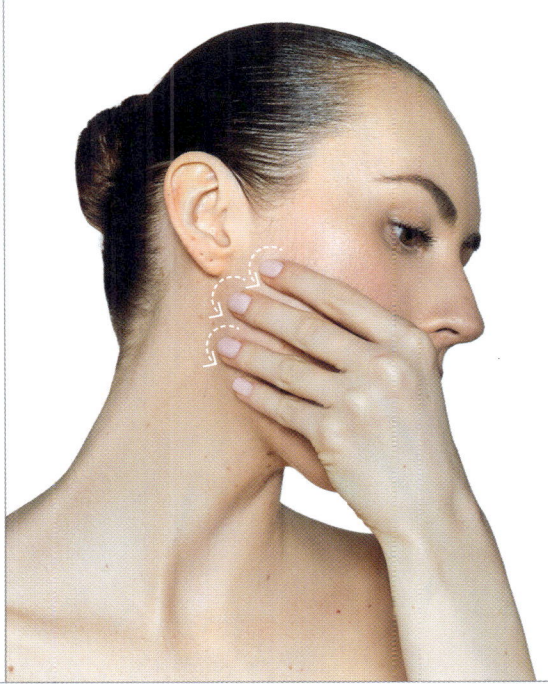

THE METHOD & MOVEMENTS

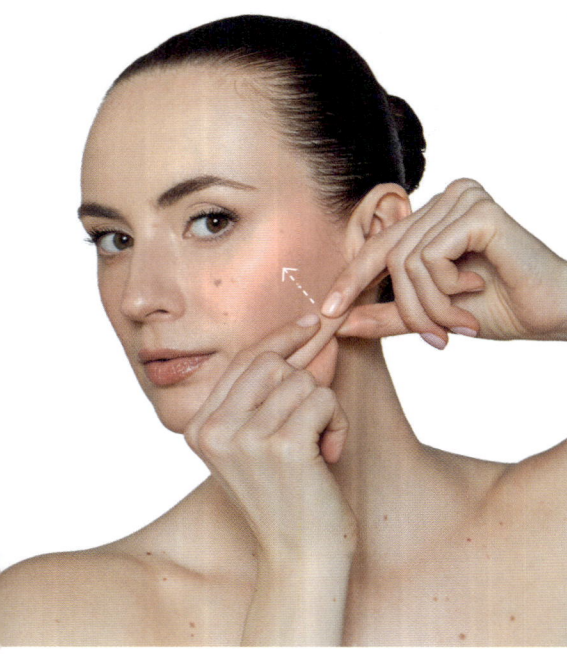

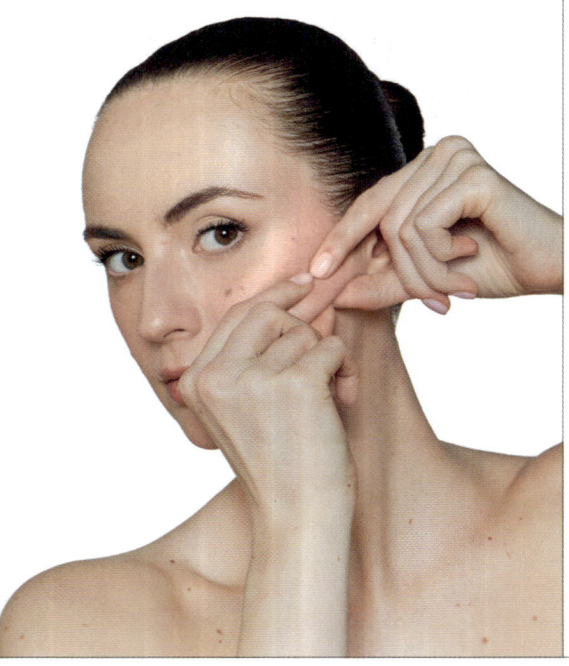

 1 MIN

The Masseter Rolls

Restore space to your lower face

This exercise softens the masseter, releases built-up tension, and reintroduces lift and mobility into the lower face. This movement is best practised without oil.

1 Grab the tissue
Using your thumbs and index fingers on both hands, gently grasp the tissue along your jawline – one hand near the ear, the other halfway between the ear and the chin. Try to hold the deeper layer of tissue, rather than just the surface skin.

2 Roll upwards
Without releasing your hold, slowly roll the tissue upwards toward the top of your cheekbones. Instead of pulling or pinching, think of lifting and stretching the underlying tissue as you glide. Keep the movement smooth, anchored, and steady. If you notice bunching near the eyes, ease the pressure slightly or use broader contact with your fingers to distribute the movement more evenly.

3 Repeat and switch
Continue rolling upwards for 30 seconds. Then switch to the other side and repeat for 30 seconds.

1 MIN

The Forehead Tap

Re-energize your skin & forehead

This exercise relaxes the upper area of your face and increases micro-blood circulation to boost the radiance of your skin and oxygen flow to the muscles in the forehead.

1 Tap
Using both hands, tap around the forehead at your own pace. You can also tap onto your scalp and around your eyes and temples. Avoid using your nails and be very gentle. You can alternate between tapping your fingers, or patting with them all at once.

2 Continue
Continue tapping for 1 minute or as long as feels nice. Don't forget to breath evenly, and relax your chest and shoulders.

> **TIP**
> *Imagine raindrops gently landing on your skin. The rhythm should be soft, never sharp. Let your fingers dance intuitively across the forehead and temples.*

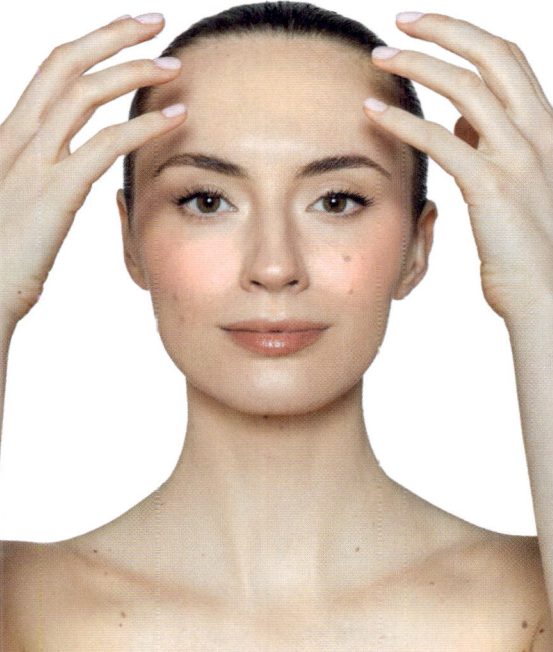
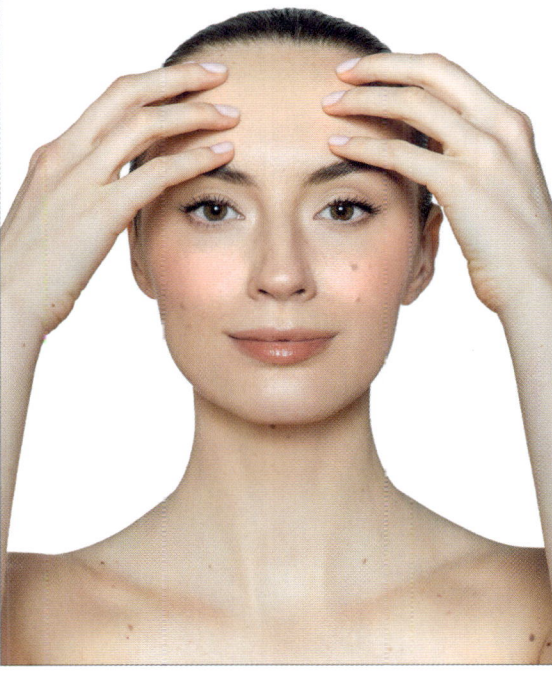

THE METHOD & MOVEMENTS

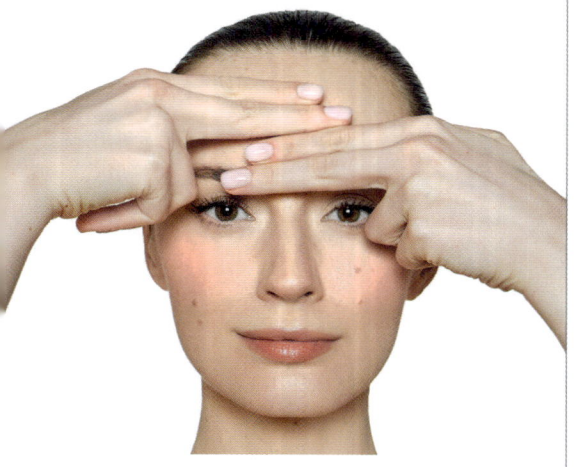

 1 MIN

The Forehead Massage

Relax overworked forehead muscles

This technique helps release tension in the forehead muscles, supporting better circulation and lymph flow. You'll want to use plenty of facial oil when doing this exercise.

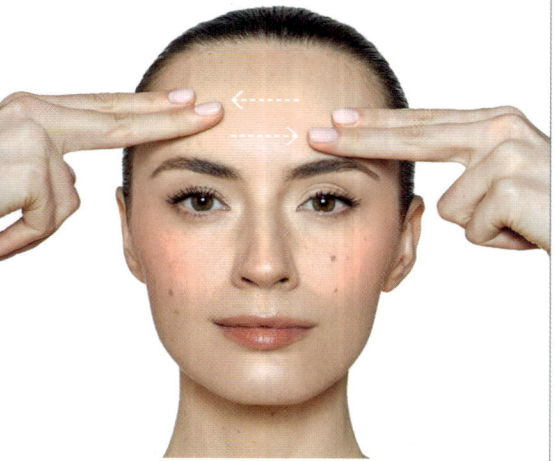

1 Place your fingers
Place your middle and ring fingers at the centre of your forehead, one hand above the other.

2 Zigzag and glide
Create a horizontal zigzag motion with both sets of fingers across your forehead, using light to medium pressure. Repeat a few times.

3 Repeat
Repeat step 2 for one minute.

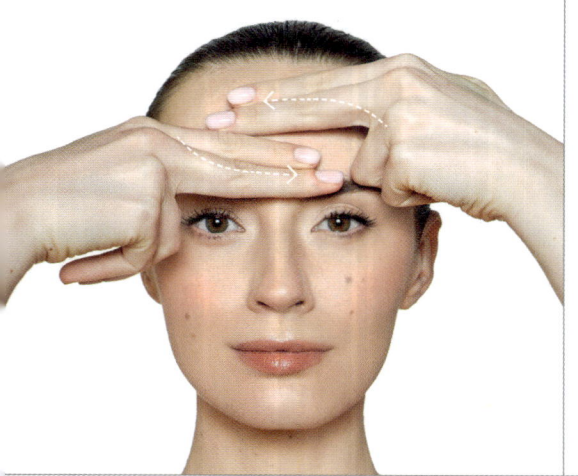

> **TIP**
> *This exercise improves the absorption of skincare, so consider adding it to your skincare daily ritual.*

1 MIN

The Forehead Knuckle Glider

Glide away tension & awaken your skin

This gliding motion releases tension in your forehead and improves micro-circulation to keep that area smooth. Don't worry if your skin goes slightly red during this exercise; just make sure you aren't causing yourself discomfort.

1 **Place your hand**
Place one hand on your hairline to gently hold the forehead taut, and in place.

2 **Glide**
Using the index knuckle on your other hand, gently glide down and up your forehead, moving from left to right.

3 **Continue**
Continue for 1 minute.

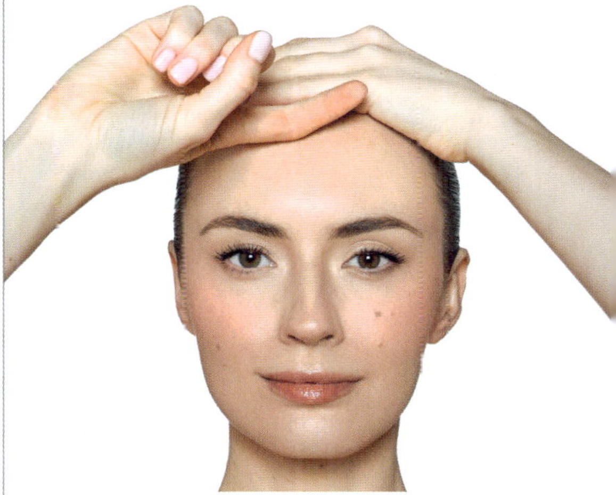

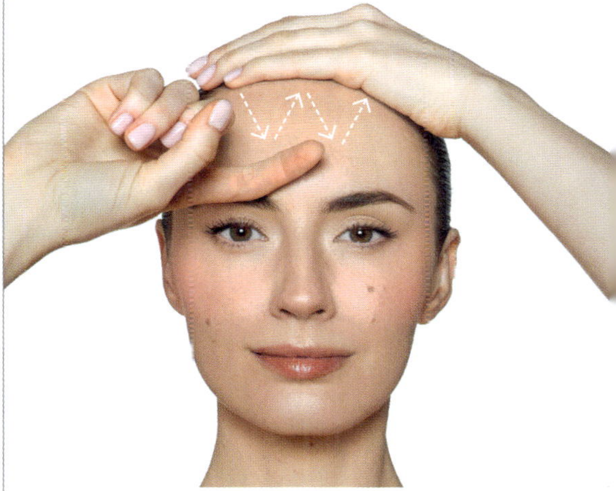

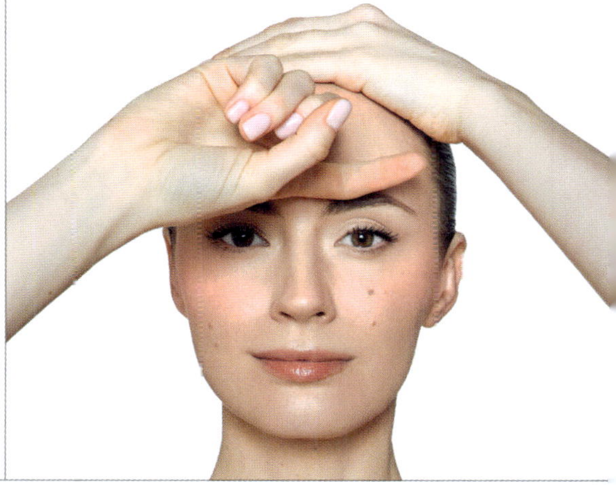

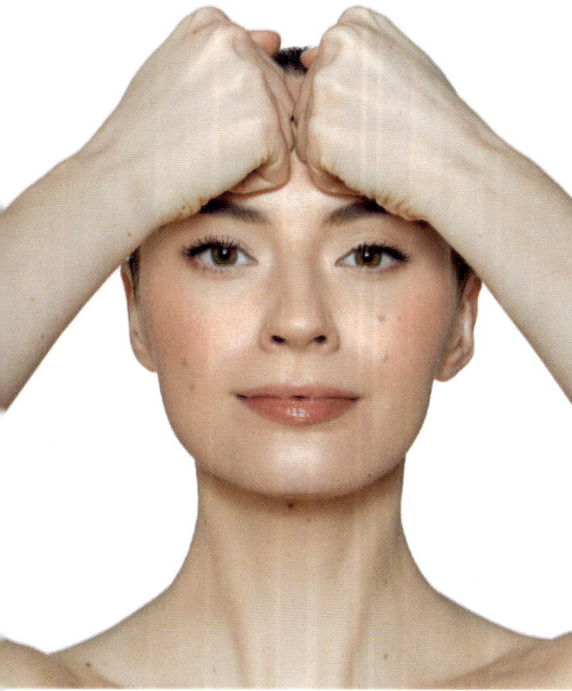

 1 MIN

The Forehead Glider

Glide away stress & soften your expression

Using a gliding motion, this exercise releases the tension in your forehead and eyebrows. Don't worry if your skin goes slightly red during this exercise; it should recover quickly.

1 Place your knuckles
Place your knuckles at the centre of your forehead.

2 Glide
Glide, but don't pull, across the forehead using medium pressure, and then down towards the temples. Hold your knuckles at the temples and create a few small circle motions. Don't forget to breathe, and keep your shoulders down.

3 Repeat
Repeat at your own pace for 1 minute, feeling the tension in your forehead melting away.

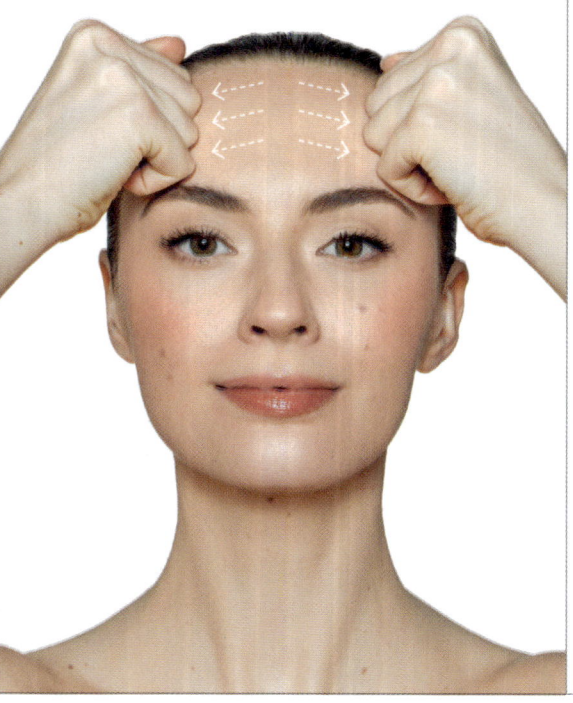

1 MIN

The Frowning X

Smooth the space between your brows

This massage technique uses your index and middle fingers to target overactive frowning muscles responsible for 11 lines. It also gently retrains facial habits that lead to expression lines.

1 Place your fingers
Place your middle and index fingers in between the eyebrows.

2 Glide
Gently glide one set of fingers diagonally across your forehead, envisaging the tension melting away. Repeat with the other hand, and alternate between the two sides to create a "X" shape. Use gentle pressure and plenty of facial oil to avoid pulling the skin.

3 Repeat
Repeat for 1 minute at your own pace, keeping your shoulders down and your face relaxed.

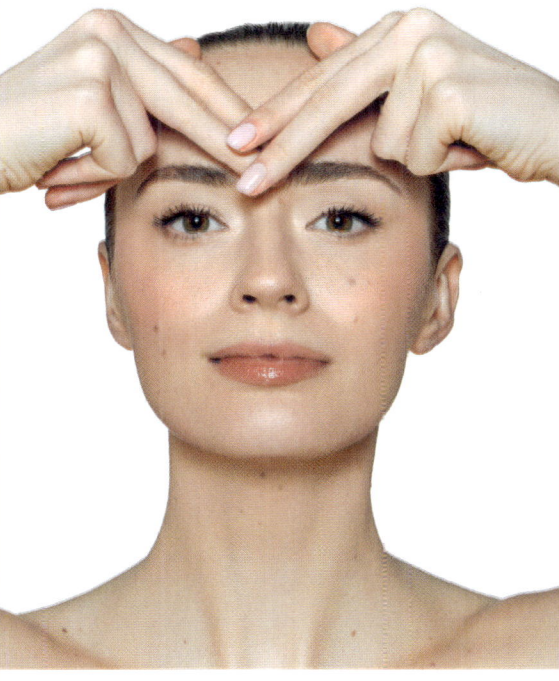

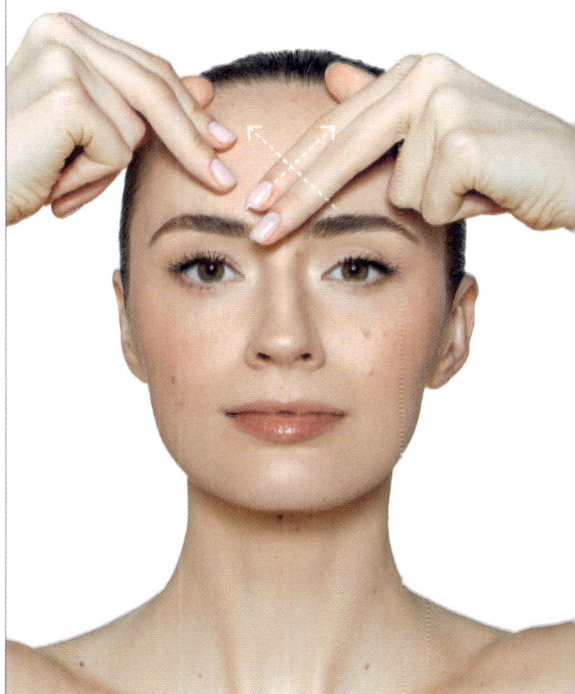

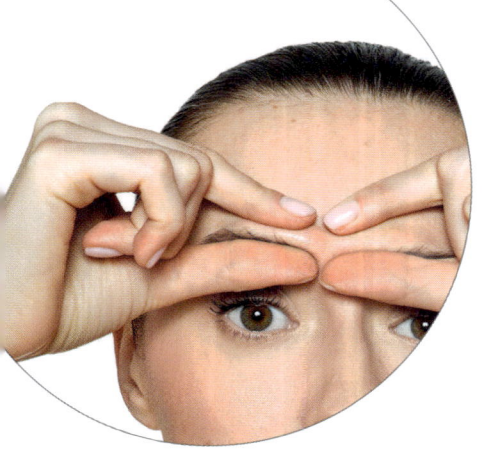

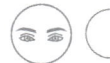 2 MIN

The 11 Line Eraser

Soften your expression & calm your mind

This exercise relaxes the overworking muscles responsible for frowning and the formation of 11 lines. It helps dissolve habitual tension, and bring softness and openness back to the upper face.

1 **Massage each eyebrow**
Gently pinch one eyebrow between both thumbs and index fingers, avoiding pulling the skin. While holding the eyebrow muscle, create a gentle circular motion to knead the muscle and release tension. Continue this pressing and massaging movement across the eyebrow for 30 seconds at a slow, even pace, keeping your shoulders relaxed.

2 **Repeat**
Repeat on the other eyebrow for 30 seconds.

3 **Massage along the brow line**
Pinch the space between your eyebrows between both thumbs and index fingers, and use the same pressing and massaging motion to move outwards towards the temples. Use each hand to work in a different direction. Continue for 1 minute.

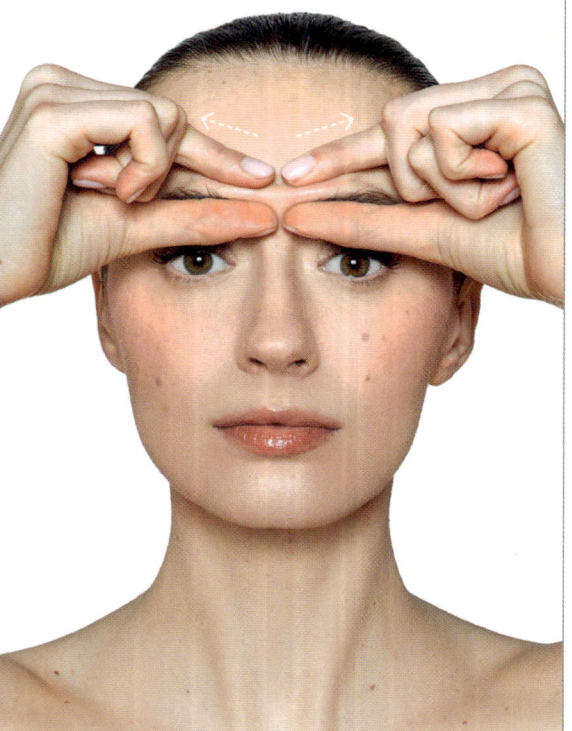

1 MIN

The Brow Lift Glide

Lift your brows & brighten your upper face

The area around your brows holds a surprising amount of tension. This technique deeply lifts the fascia beneath the skin to support smoother forehead movement.

> **TIP**
> This is one of the best techniques to refresh tired eyes and reduce expression lines, and is best done without oil.

1 Anchor the brow
Place both index fingers horizontally above one eyebrow.

2 Glide and lift
Together, glide the fingers upwards from just above the brow towards the hairline in a slow, deep stroke. The movement should be slow, intentional, and deep.

3 Repeat and switch
Repeat the glide in the same area for 30 seconds, then switch sides and repeat for another 30 seconds. Feel how the area becomes softer and more mobile.

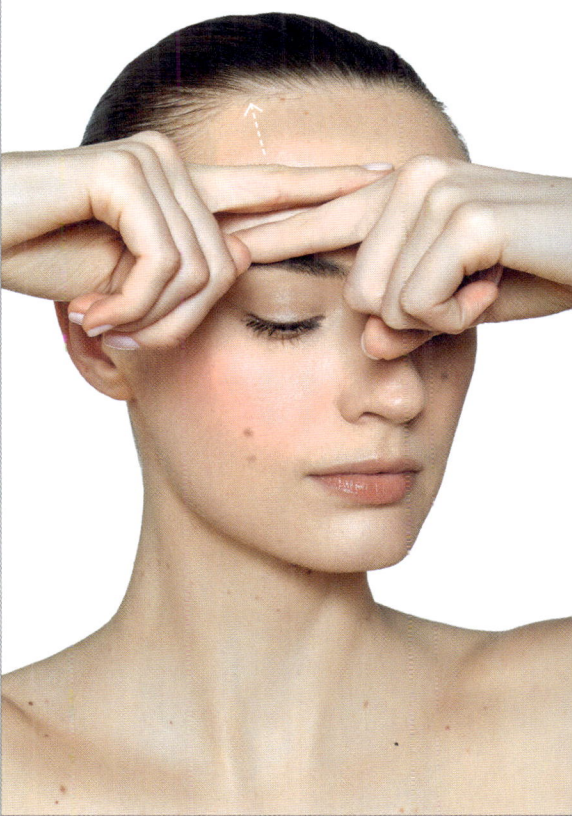

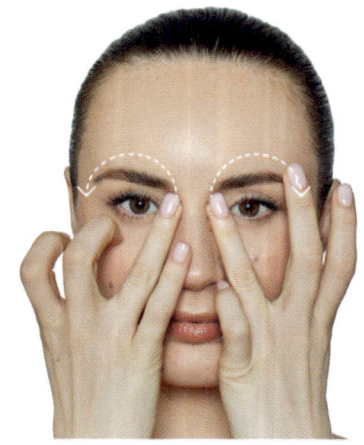

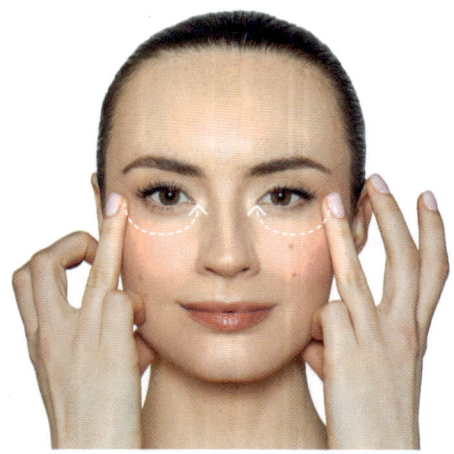

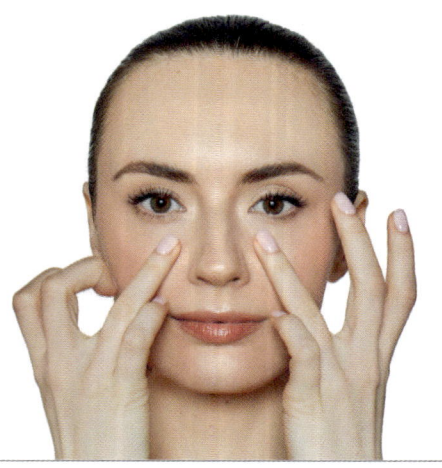

 1 MIN

The Eye Massage

Calm & brighten your eye area

This gentle eye massage improves blood circulation, lymphatic drainage, and collagen stimulation in the eye area, which can help reduce puffiness, soften fine lines, and relieve tension.

1 **Massage around your eyes**
Place your ring fingers gently into the inner eye corners, and create gentle circular motions around the eye, gliding up and above the eyebrow, then down and across the under eye.

2 **Repeat**
Repeat these circles for 1 minute at your own pace, closing your eyes if you'd prefer.

1 MIN

The Upper Eyelid Depuffer

Awaken & depuff your eyes

This massage stimulates lymphatic drainage around the eyes, and refreshes the entire upper face. It's especially beneficial in the mornings or after screen-heavy days.

1 Place your thumbs
Press your thumbs under the inner corners of your eyebrows. You will feel a hollow notch here called the supraorbital notch.

2 Glide
Using light pressure, glide your thumbs right under your eyebrow bone to move any unnecessary lymph fluid out of your eyelids. You can also place your index fingers on your forehead to help maintain the gentle pressure of the glide.

3 Repeat
Continue at your own pace for 1 minute.

TIP
Let your thumbs follow the contour of your brow bone like a soft windshield wiper – slow, smooth, and steady. Avoid pressing into the eyelid or dragging the skin.

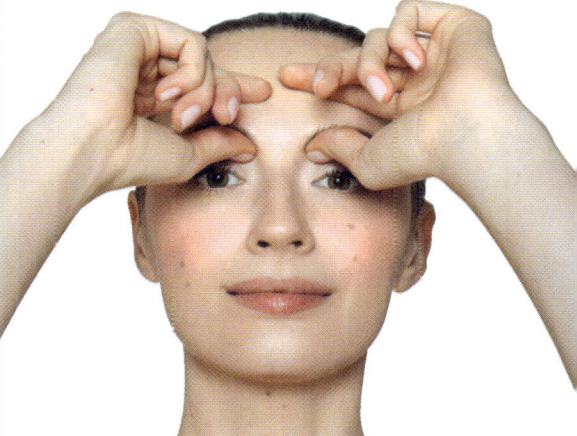

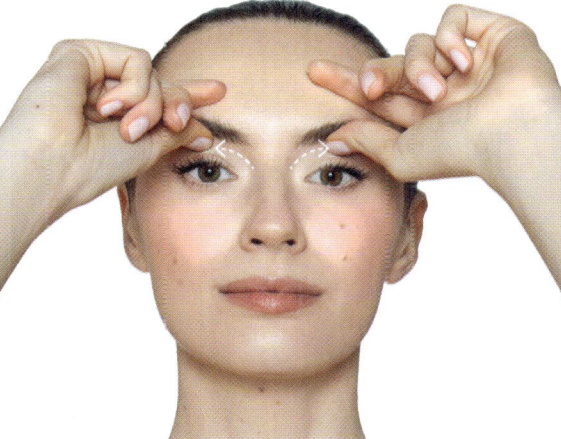

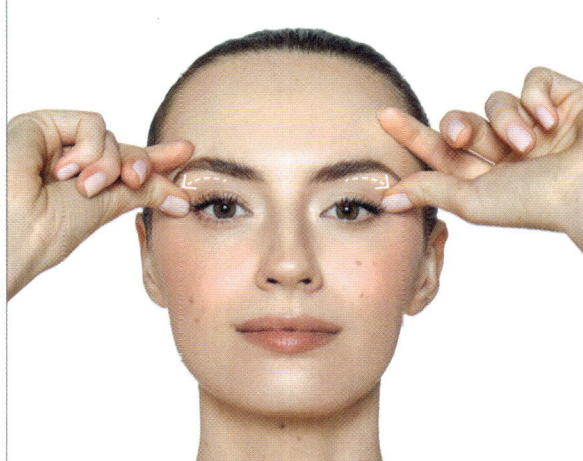

THE METHOD & MOVEMENTS

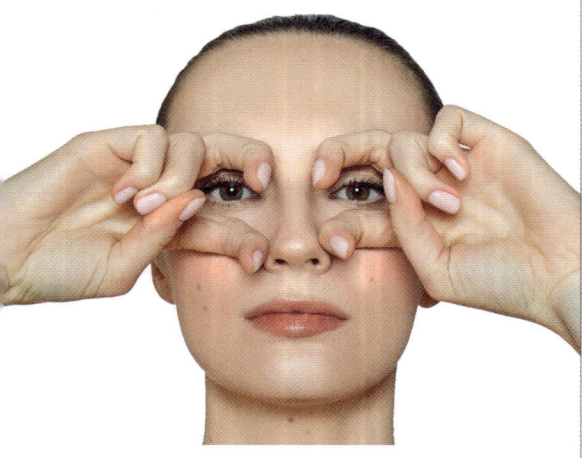
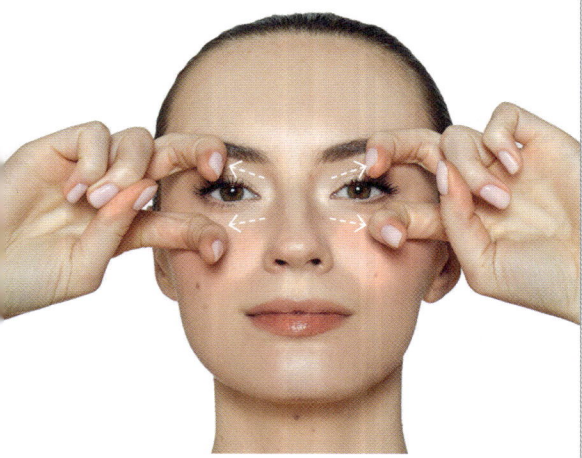
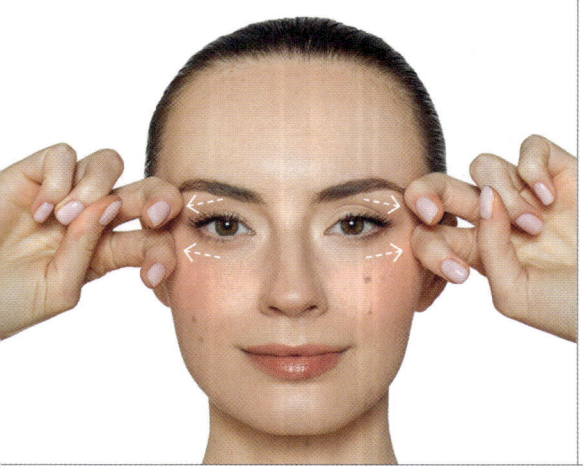

 1 MIN

The Eye Knuckle Glider

Sweep away stagnation & soothe eyes

This exercise releases tension from the eyes. The knuckle glide stimulates circulation, encourages fluid movement, and can help signs of fatigue, especially after screen time, stress, or lack of sleep.

1 **Place your knuckles**
Place your index and middle knuckles towards the inner eye corners, with the middle knuckle resting on the eyebrow, and the index knuckles resting on the under-eye.

2 **Glide**
Glide the knuckles across the eyes until you get to the tail far end of your eyebrows. Wiggle at the temples. You can avoid wrinkling the skin by using enough facial oil.

3 **Continue**
Continue the movement for 1 minute at your own pace.

2 MIN

The Eye Depuffer

Refresh & reset tired eyes

This exercise is a great way to depuff and relax the entire eye area by pressing four key acupressure points. It supports lymphatic flow, reduces stagnation, and brings clarity to the upper face.

1 Depuff the upper eyes
Place your thumbs into the notch under your eyebrow, at the inner corner of the eye, and your index fingers on your forehead for support. Apply firm pressure into the thumbs for 30 seconds without pulling at the skin. Then, lift your fingers and move to the middle upper eye area, beneath your eyebrow bone. Press for 30 seconds.

2 Depuff the side of the eyes
Use your index fingers to press firmly into the corners of your eyes, right at the bone. Hold for 30 seconds.

3 Depuff the under-eyes
Using your index finger, press into the eye socket right underneath the eyes. Apply medium pressure here, as the skin beneath your eyes is very delicate. Hold for 30 seconds. Finally, move to the inner corners of your eye, apply pressure, and hold for 30 seconds.

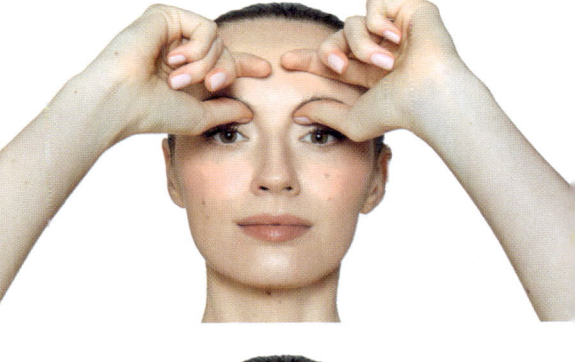
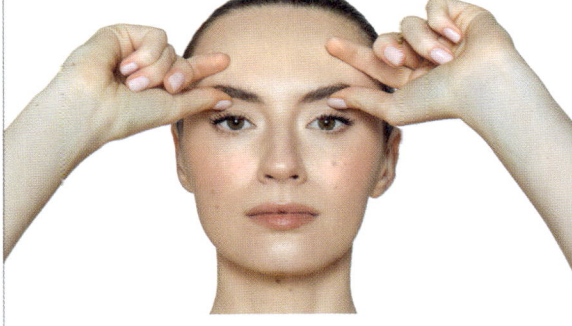
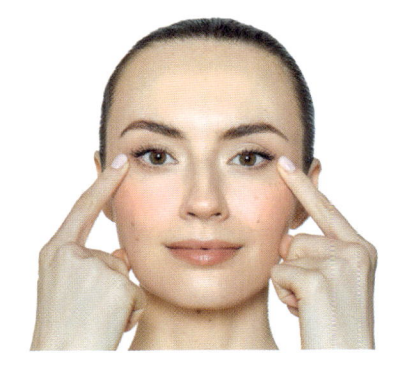
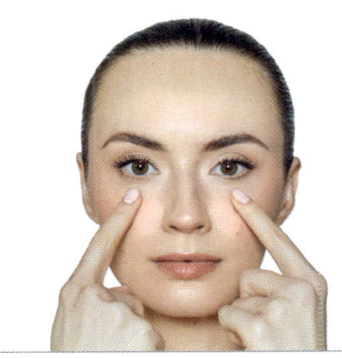

THE METHOD & MOVEMENTS

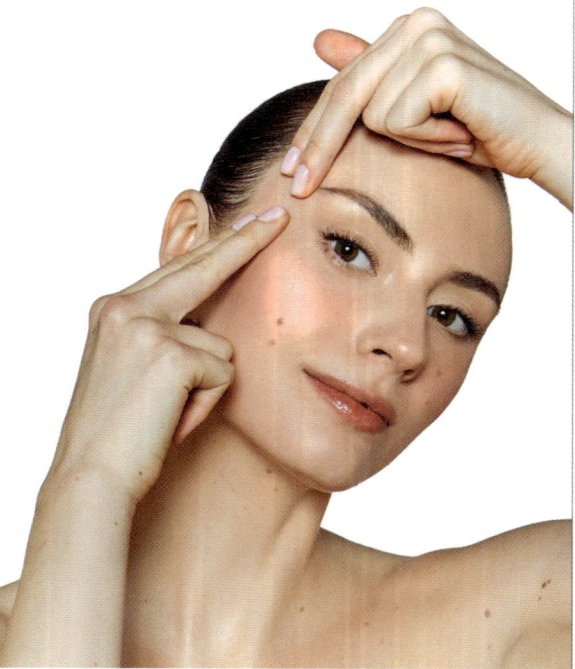

 1 MIN

The Crow's Feet Release

Soften tight eye corners

The area around the outer eyes often holds tension, contributing to tightness and fine lines known as crow's feet. This glide helps restore gentleness, hydration, and elasticity to this expressive zone.

1 Place your fingers
Place the fingertips of your left index and middle finger of one hand just above the crow's feet (near the temple) next to your right eye, and the right index and middle fingertips just below the outer corner of the right eye, along the cheekbone.

2 Stretch in opposite directions
Gently glide the top hand upwards towards the hairline, while the bottom hand glides downwards and slightly out towards the jaw. This creates a subtle inside-out stretch, lengthening the muscles and loosening tight fascia.

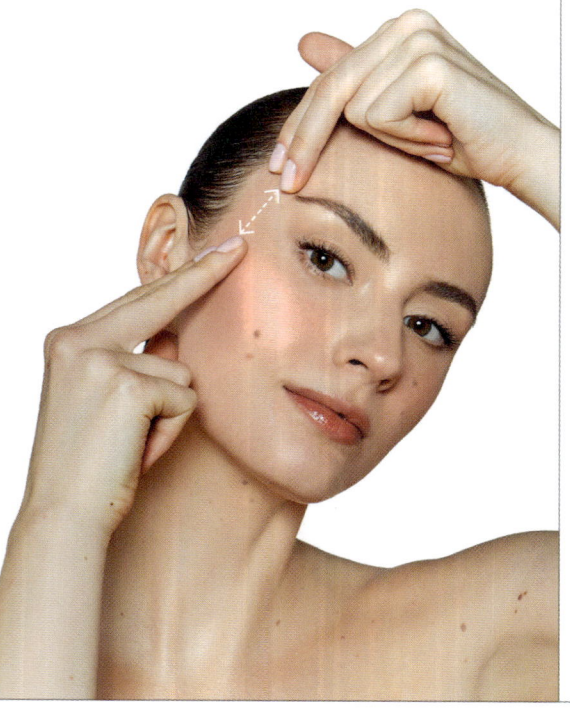

3 Move with control
Repeat this gliding motion slowly and with awareness for 30 seconds at your own pace. Pause if you feel resistance, and use your breath to stay present and relaxed.

4 Switch and finish
Repeat on the other side for 30 seconds.

4-6 REPS

The Under-Eye Zigzag

Reduce puffiness in tired eyes

The delicate under-eye area is often one of the first places to show signs of stress or fatigue. This motion helps to restore a soft, open look to your eyes. You'll want to use oil for this move.

1. Place your fingers
Place the sides of your index fingers gently under your eyes, just above the orbital bone (see page 31) towards the inner corners of your eye.

2. Zigzag outwards
Begin to glide your fingers outwards along the contour of the orbital bone, moving towards the temples in a small zigzag pattern. Think of drawing tiny diagonal lines or making quick mini upside-down "V" shapes, shifting slightly up and down as you move sideways. The movement should be gentle, light, and continuous, like tracing a soft wave.

3. Repeat and finish
Practise the second step 2–3 times on each side of the face.

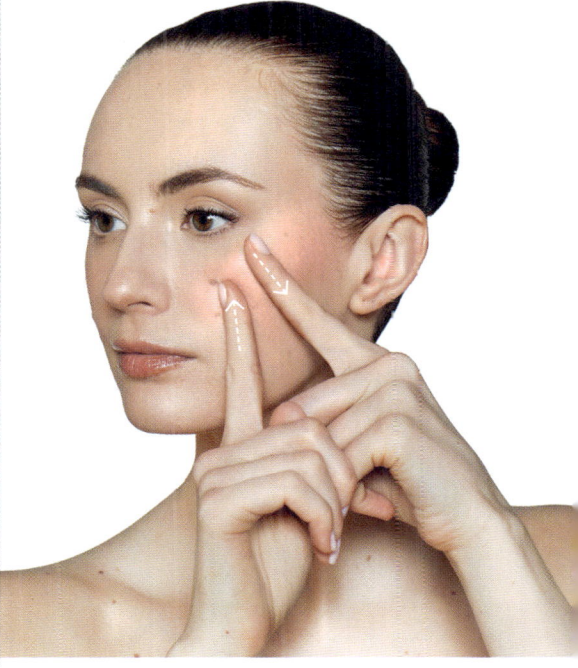

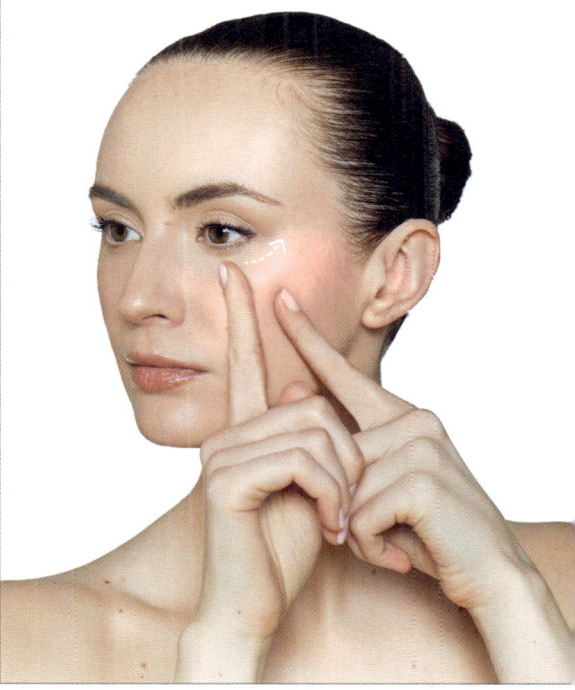

THE METHOD & MOVEMENTS

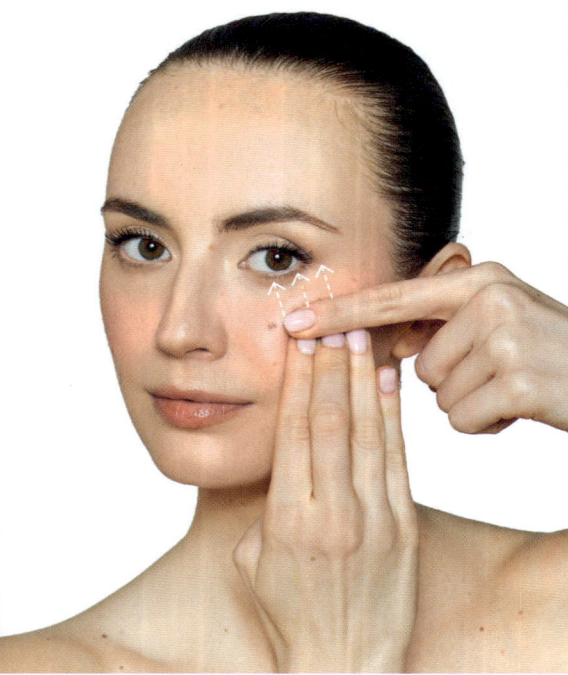
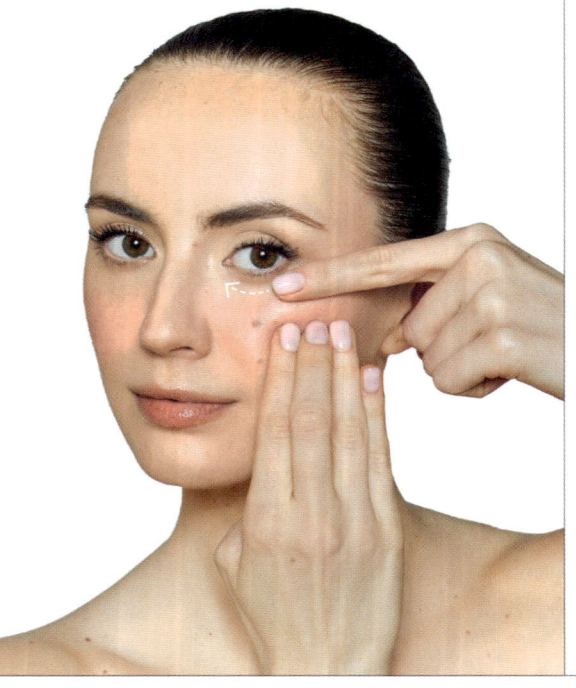

 4-6 REPS

The Hollow Eye Lift

Support fullness & refresh beneath your eyes

This fascia lift technique targets the orbicularis oculi muscle in the under-eye area, helping to rehydrate, release, and support a fuller, brigther look beneath the eyes.

1 **Anchor the muscle**
Press the index, middle, and ring finger on your right hand gently into the tissue beneath the orbital bone on your left eye, so that your index finger is beneath the outer corner of the eye. Keep your pressure light but steady, without pushing into the eye socket.

2 **Lift vertically**
With the index finger of your left hand placed horizontally above your anchored fingers, lift the fascia straight up towards the lower edge of the eye – not diagonally – using slow, mini-glides. Repeat this motion 2-3 times to encourage gentle release.

3 **Work along the under-eye**
Move laterally along the orbital bone in small sections, gliding from the outer to the inner corner of the eye. Repeat 2-3 times.

4 **Switch sides**
Move to the other eye and follow the same steps.

6-10 REPS

The Eye Roll Lift

Lift & awaken tired eyes in seconds

This fascia roll gently lifts and resets the tissue around your eyes, softening expression and awakening the upper face. This is a perfect to do before applying eye cream or makeup.

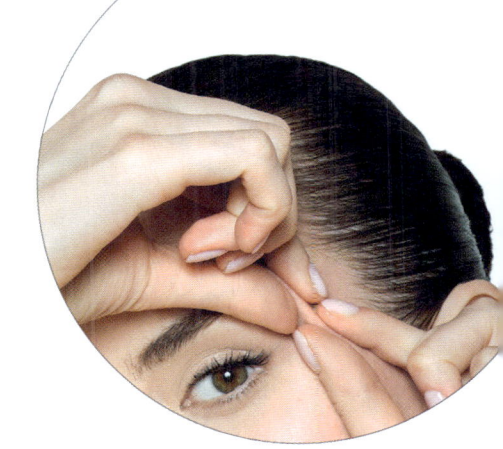

1 Grab the tissue
Gently hold the tissue at the outer corner of one eye with between your thumbs and index fingers, so that your top hand is pinching just beneath the tail end of your eyebrow, angling up towards your forehead, and your other hand is pinching just beneath it, elbow pointing down towards the floor. It may help to move your head to one side while doing this exercise.

2 Roll diagonally upwards
Without letting go of the tissue, begin to glide it diagonally up towards your temple and outer hairline. Focus on lifting and smoothing the deeper layer beneath the skin, rather than dragging the surface. If you notice the skin above your fingers wrinkling or bunching, try widening your grip slightly or easing your pressure to create more glide with less drag.

3 Repeat and switch sides
Repeat the roll 3-5 times on one side, then repeat on the other side for the same number of repetitions.

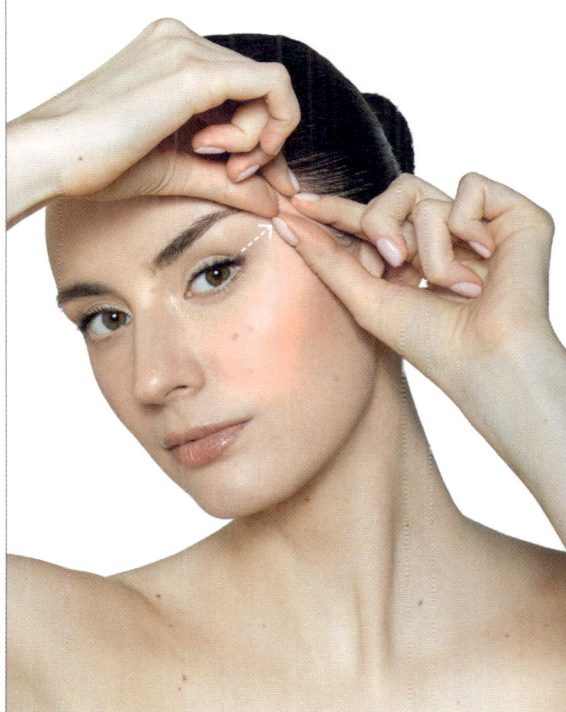

THE METHOD & MOVEMENTS

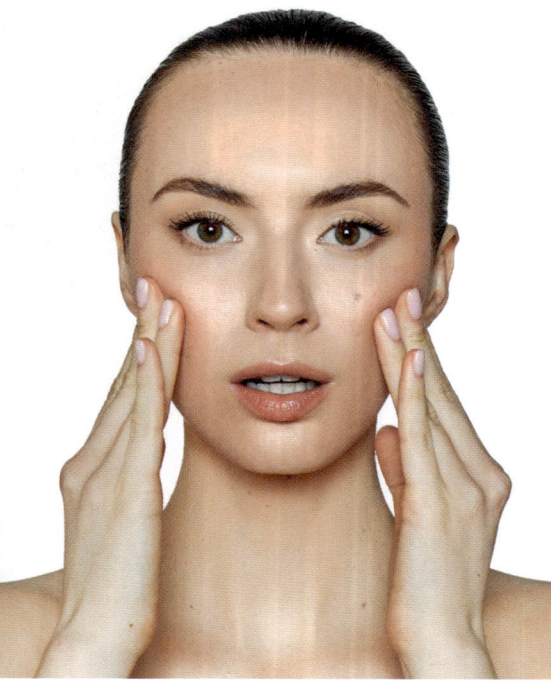

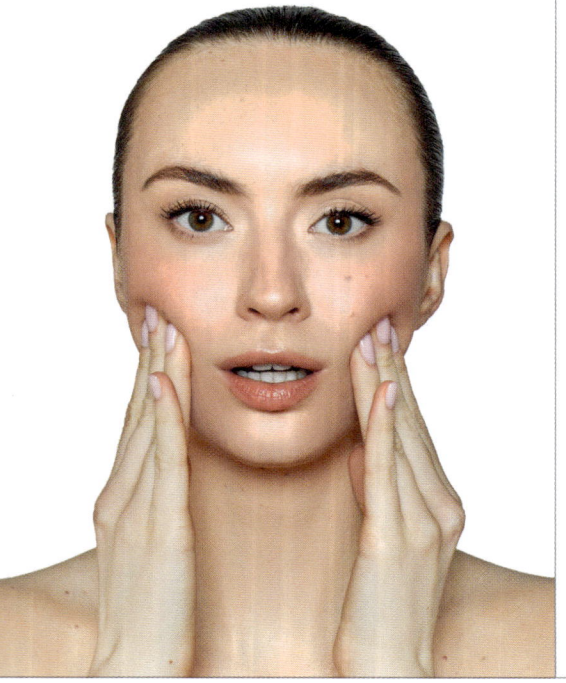

 1.5 MIN

The Cheek Relaxer

Release tension from your cheeks & jaw

This exercise unwinds tightness in your mid-face area. It's ideal for decompressing after a long day, helping reduce tightness from clenching and restoring volume and softness to the centre-face.

1   **Press your cheeks**
Press your index, middle, and ring fingers into the apples of your cheek. Alternatively, you can use your knuckles for more intensity. Hold for 30 seconds, using whatever pressure feels right for you.

2   **Press your jawline**
Move down and press your three fingers or knuckles into the jawline. Hold for 30 seconds, using whatever pressure feels right for you.

3   **Press under your cheekbones**
Finally, press your three fingers or knuckles into the space beneath your cheekbones for 30 seconds, feeling the tension release.

1 MIN

The Nasolabial Fold Eraser

Soften & smooth out smile lines

This exercise releases tension that is usually responsible for nasolabial folds. It's normal if your skin becomes a little red here; just make sure you aren't causing yourself any discomfort.

1 Place your fingers
Place your index fingers or knuckles next to your nostrils.

2 Circle
Gently massage in small circular motions for 30 seconds at a firm pressure.

3 Move up
Move your index fingers up and down the sides of the nose, slowly continuing to massage in small circular motions using medium to deep pressure for 30 seconds.

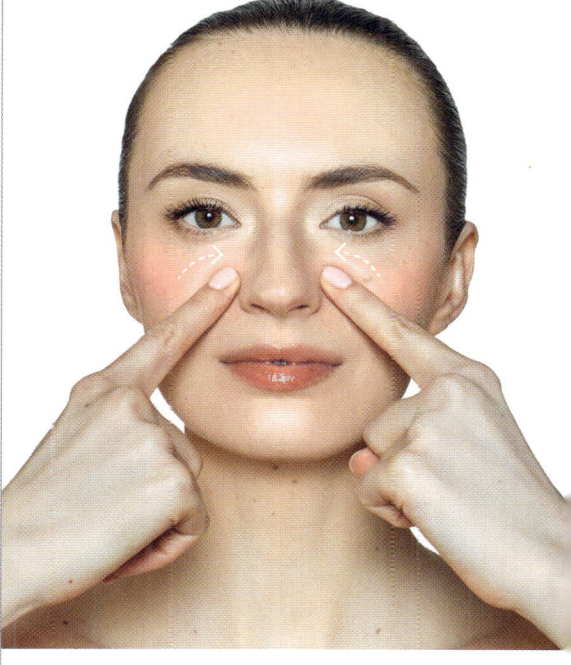

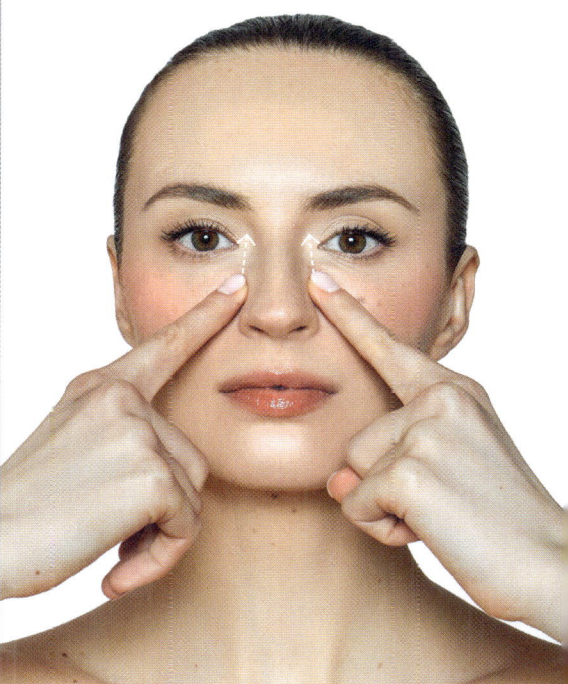

THE METHOD & MOVEMENTS

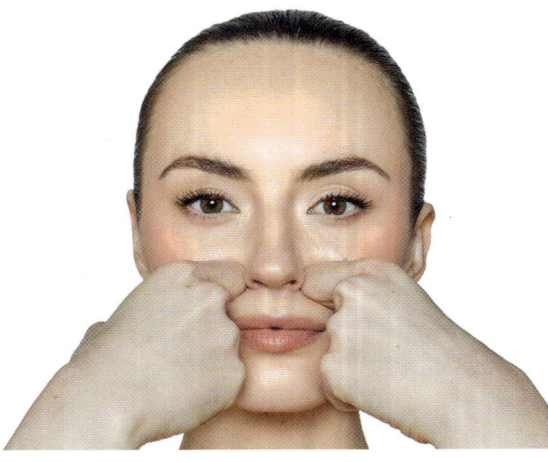
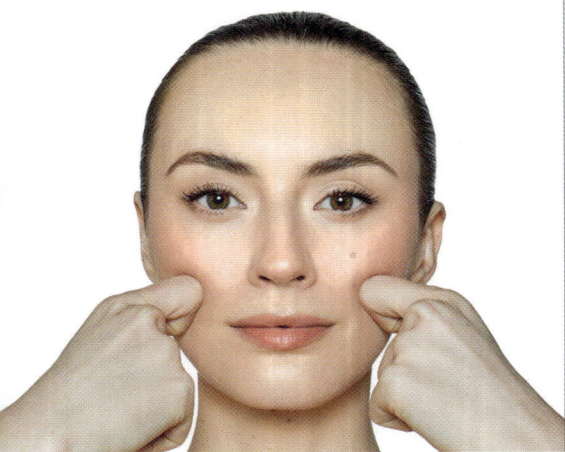
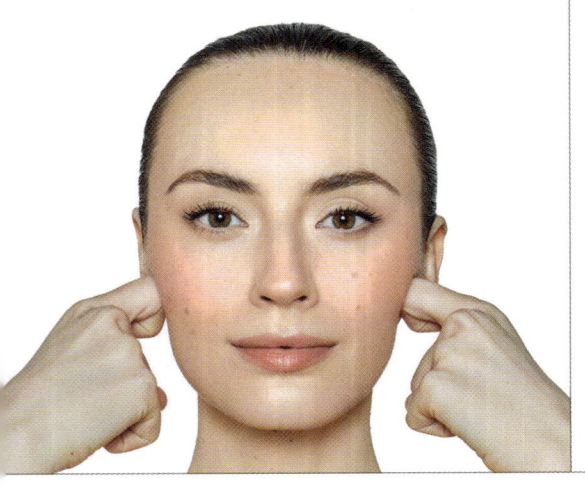

 1.5 MIN

The Cheekbone Sculpt

Awaken & define your cheekbones

This exercise relieves tension, helping to improve blood flow and ease muscular tightness. It's especially helpful for defining and refreshing facial contours and softening smile lines.

1 Press next to your nose
Place your index fingers or knuckles next to your nostrils. Gently apply firm pressure for 30 seconds, melting away tension. You can also massage the area using little circular motions.

2 Press your cheekbones
Next, press your index knuckles firmly under your cheeks. Hold for 30 seconds, incorporating small circular motions if it feels right to you.

3 Press towards your ears
Finally, press your index fingers or knuckles firmly towards the end of your cheekbone, right next to the ears, feeling the tension release. Hold for 30 seconds, wiggling in circular motions if you choose.

1 MIN

The Cheek Glider

Smooth, sculpt, & soften the cheeks

This massage releases tension stored and supports lymphatic drainage, helping to reduce puffiness and soften deep expression lines. It also encourages a lifted, refreshed appearance.

1 Press
Press your palms into your nasolabial folds.

2 Glide
Glide with medium pressure diagonally across your cheek muscles, and up towards your ears and temples. Avoid wrinkling your skin and use more facial oil to help with the gliding motion.

3 Repeat
Repeat this movement evenly and slowly for 1 minute, envisaging releasing tension from your nasolabial folds and cheeks.

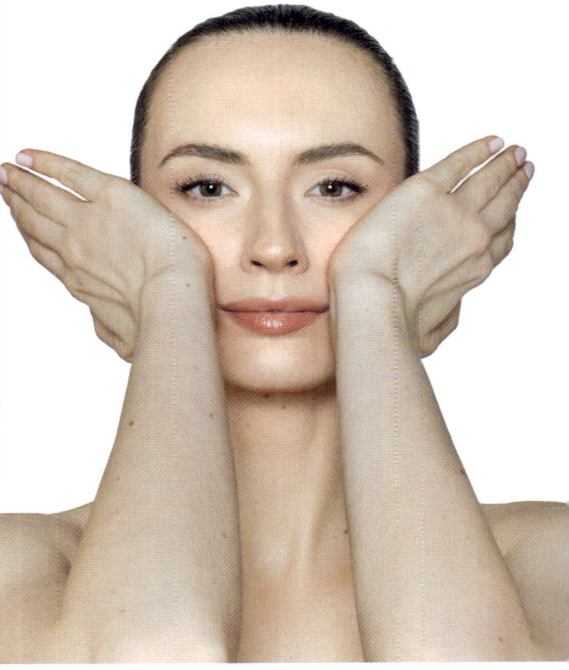
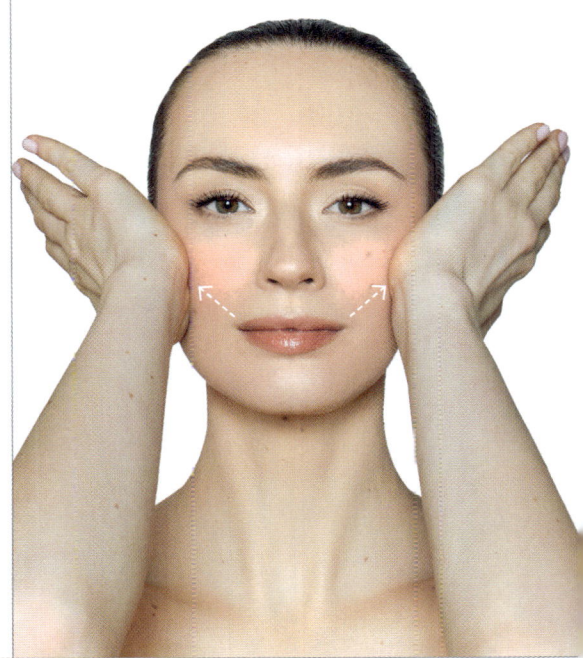

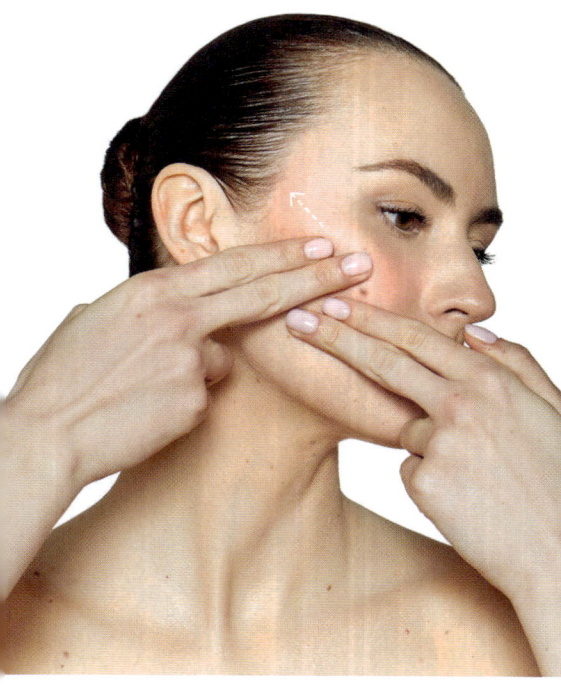

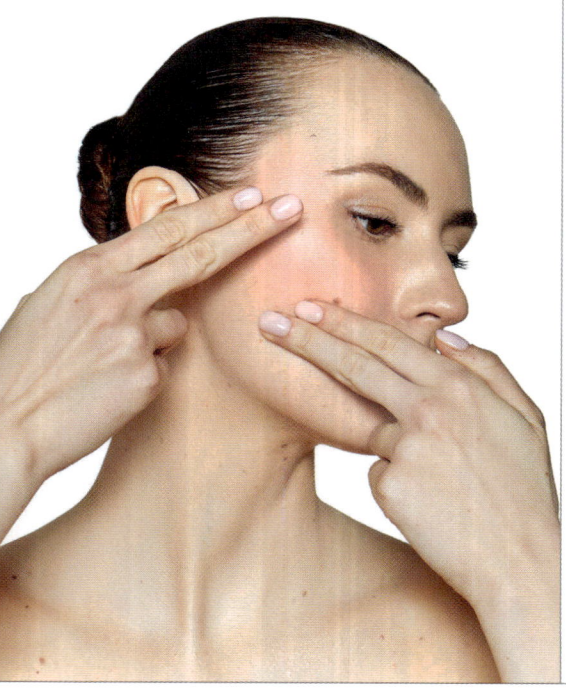

 1 MIN

The Cheek Flick

Wake up dull skin & energize your cheeks

This exercise improves blood circulation to give you dewy, rosy, and lifted cheeks. It helps brighten your complexion, which is perfect before makeup or as a mid-day refresh.

1 Place your fingers
Place your index and middle fingers on one nasolabial fold to hold your skin steady, and act as an anchor.

2 Flick the top hand
Use the other hand to gently flick up and out on the cheek using the middle and index fingertips. Flick quickly, rhythmically, and evenly, being careful not to tug the skin. Keep the other hand anchored, and continue for 30 seconds.

3 Repeat
Repeat on the other side for 30 seconds.

> **TIP**
> *Keep your movements light and snappy, like you're tapping a drum. The rhythm is what boosts the flow, not heavy pressure.*

1 MIN

The Cheekbone Definer

TIP

Think of your hand as a shelf and your head as a heavy fruit – let it gently sink without forcing anything. The still pressure is what creates the release.

Define by releasing tension & puffiness

By allowing the weight of your head to melt into your hand in this exercise, this movement helps define the cheekbones, reduce puffiness, and improve muscle tone in a subtle yet effective way.

1 Place your hand
Create an "L" shape with your left hand, and rest the back of the hand against the contour of your left cheekbone, right into the muscle.

2 Relax your head
Relax the weight of your head into your hand to feel the tension release, pressing slightly into the hand. Try not to slouch forwards, and keep your shoulders down and relaxed. Hold for 30 seconds.

3 Repeat
Repeat on the other side for 30 seconds.

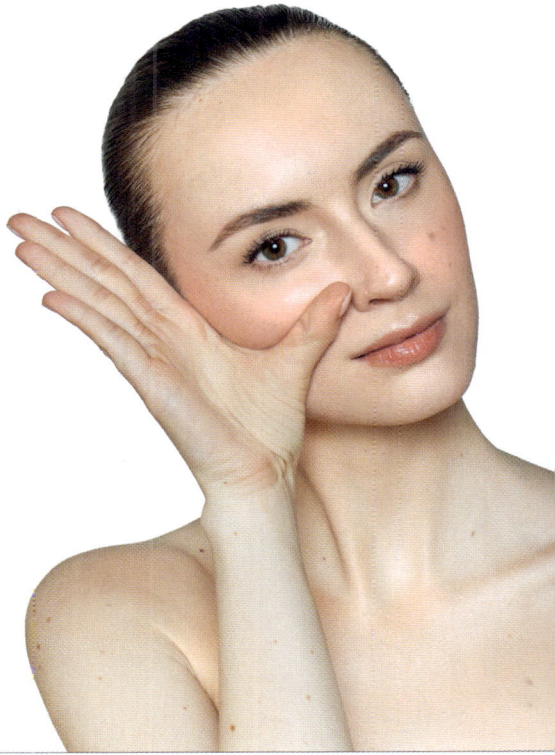

THE METHOD & MOVEMENTS

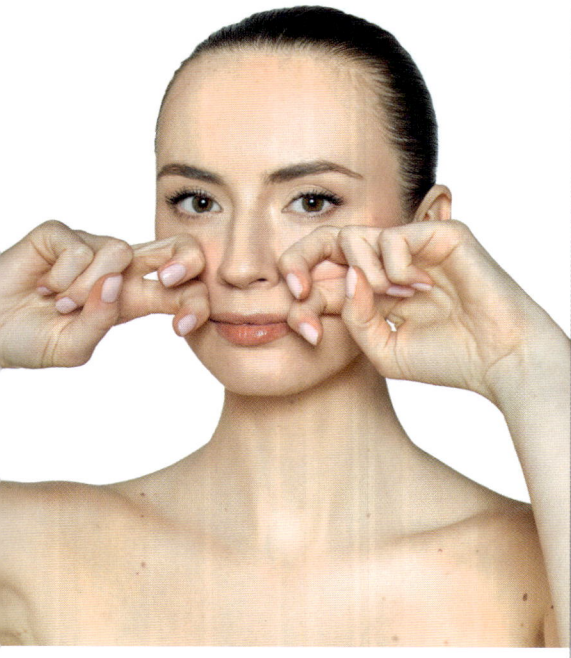
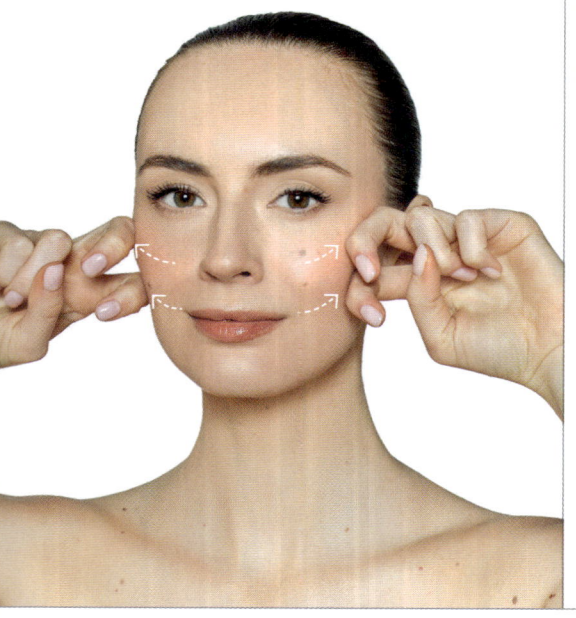

 1 MIN

The Midi Cheek Sculpter

Lift, sculpt, & energize your cheeks

This sculpting motion is a great way to depuff, tone, and shape the mid part of your face. It also helps relax facial tension and promotes a more defined, lifted appearance over time.

1 **Place your knuckles**
Place your index and middle knuckles on either side of your nose.

2 **Glide**
Glide evenly across your cheeks towards your ears, placing your knuckles right around the cheekbones and wiggling slightly at the end of the motion, towards the ears. Use medium pressure, avoid dragging or wrinkling the skin, and imagine yourself sculpting your face. Repeat for 1 minute, feeling the lymph fluid moving out of your face.

> **TIP**
> *Use just enough pressure to feel the tissue shift under your skin – like you're gently shaping clay, not pushing hard.*

FACE YOGA

1 MIN

The Mouth Relaxer

Let go of mouth & facial tension

This pose is great for relaxing the muscles around the mouth, as it helps to release built-up tension from speaking, clenching, or facial workouts.

1 **Blow out through your mouth**
Take a deep breath, and then blow the air out heavily through your mouth. Allow your lips to vibrate and make a "Brrrrrrrrrrr" sound.

2 **Repeat**
Continue this exercise for 1 minute, taking deep breaths in between each exhale.

TIP
To help with this movement, imagine you are imitating a horse, just like we do when we are children. Let your lips ripple and your breath flow naturally. It's all about release, not control.

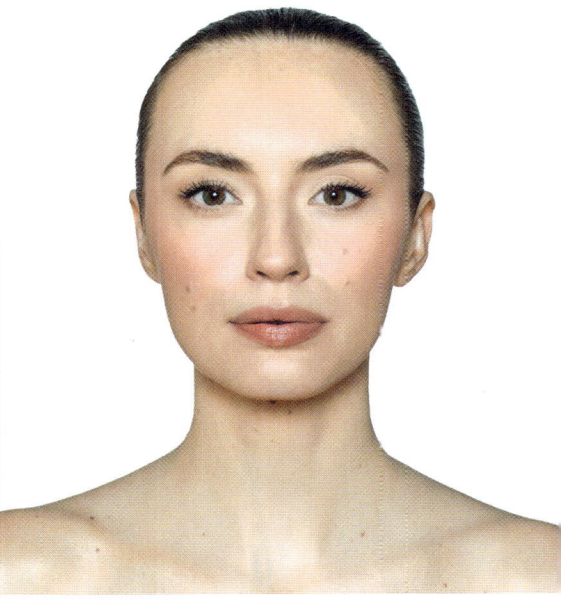

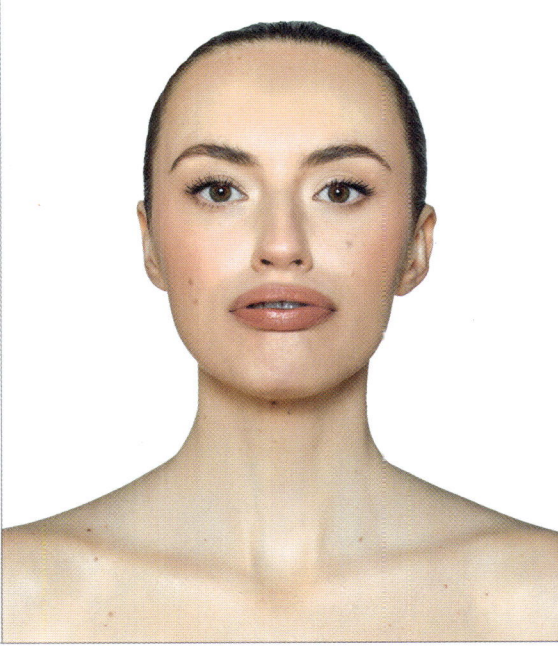

THE METHOD & MOVEMENTS

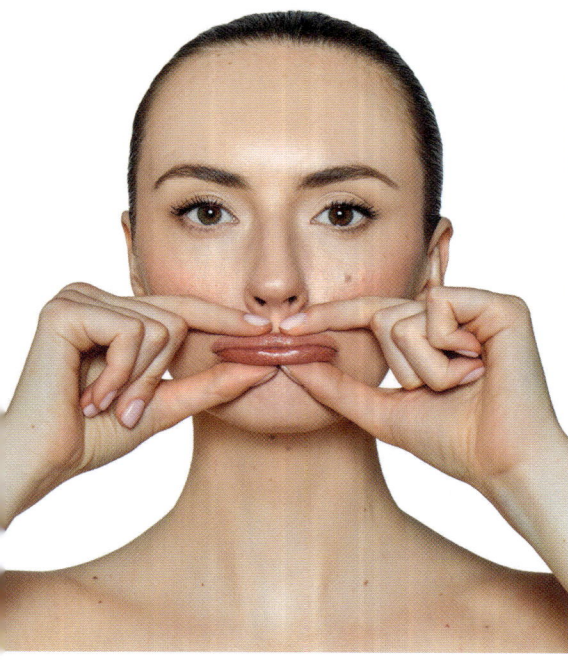

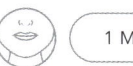 1 MIN

The Pouty Lip

Plump, smooth, & soften your lips

This exercise plumps your lips, boosts collagen production, and relaxes the circular muscle around the mouth. It also helps soften the edges of the lips, where habitual clenching often accumulates.

1 **Place your fingers**
Gently hold your mouth between your index fingers and thumbs.

2 **Press**
Firmly press into the tissue and shake the section of mouth from side to side. Release the fingers, move across the mouth, and grab another section. Repeat the press and shake.

3 **Continue**
Continue for one minute, moving across the entire mouth and back, staying relaxed and massaging the tension away. Pay special attention to the very edges of the mouth, which includes the cheeks, as we hold a lot of tension here.

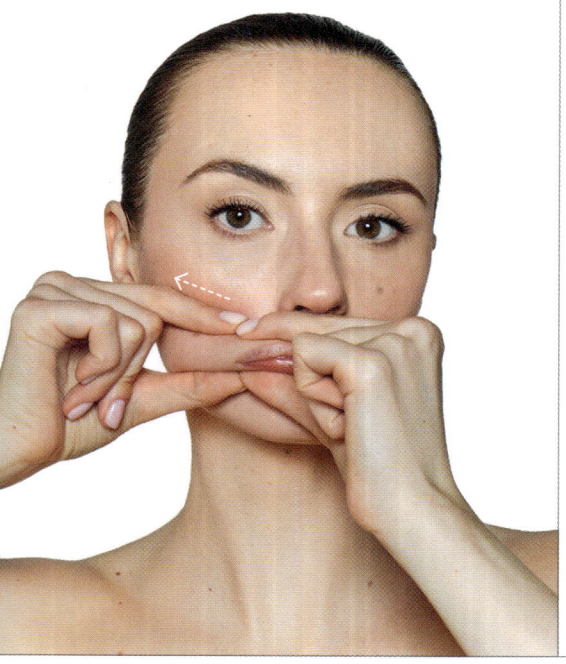

TIP
Use slow, intentional pressure – like you're gently pressing tension out of the lips. Be especially mindful at the corners, where tightness can pull the lips downwards over time.

1 MIN

The Lip Liner

Enhance your natural lip shape

This exercises helps contour the lips and make them appear more plump. It increases micro-circulation in the lips and supports tone in the surrounding muscles that maintain your lip line.

1 Pinch
Gently pinch along the contours of your lip line with your thumbs and index fingers, beginning at the middle of the top lip. Use both hands so that they are moving away from one another, and move from the inner to the outer parts of the lip. Move to the lower lip and pinch at your own pace, working your way from the centre of the lip to the edges, with both hands pinching along the same side. Make sure you gently pinch the lips rather than pulling the skin, imagining you're pressing a button.

2 Continue
Continue for 1 minute, staying relaxed.

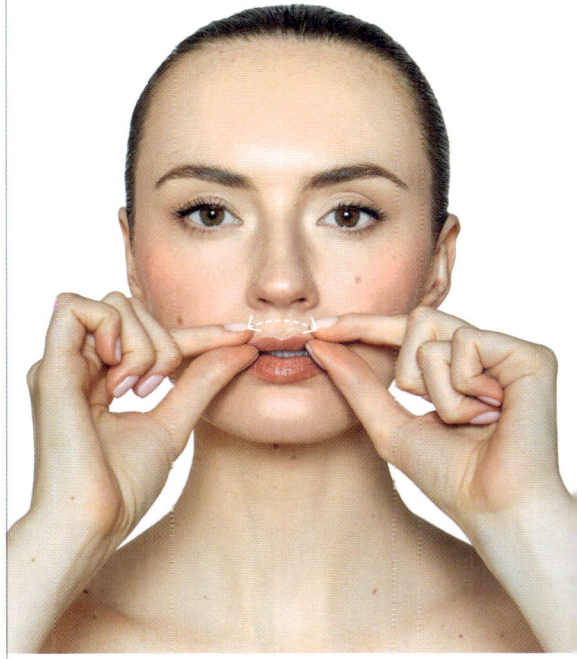

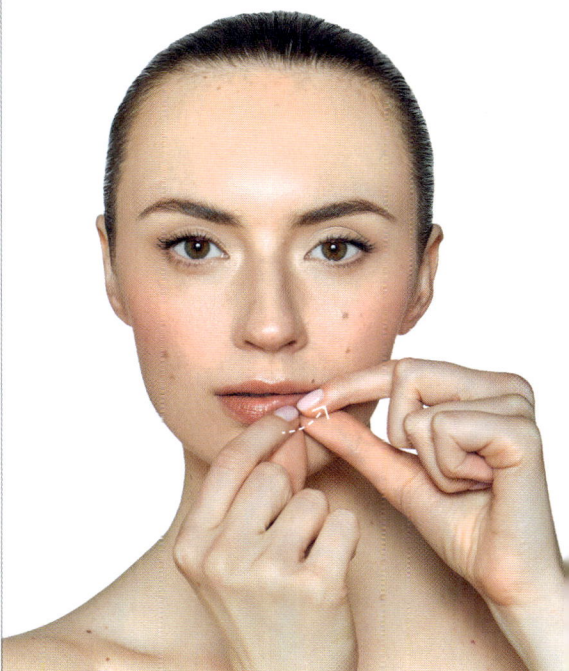

THE METHOD & MOVEMENTS

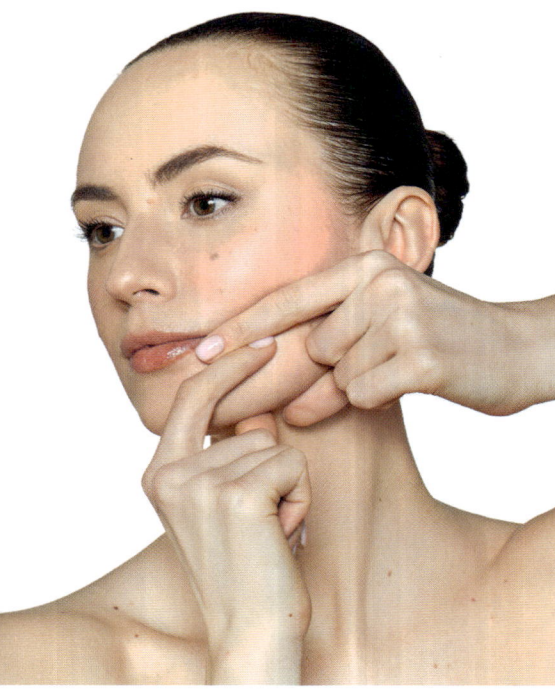
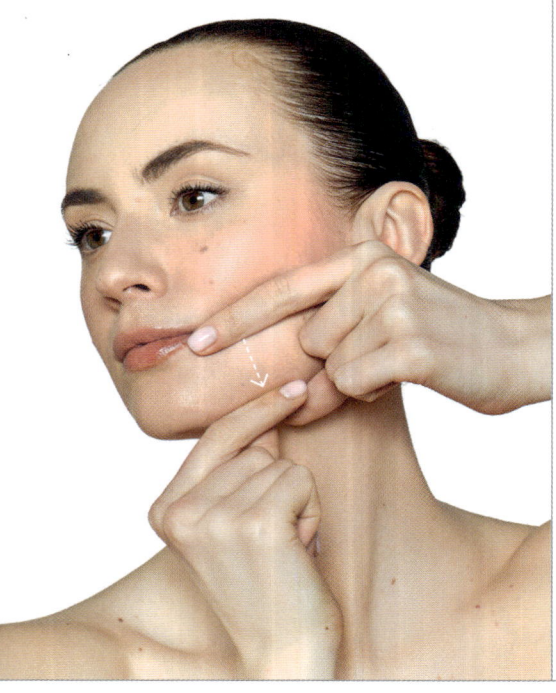

 6-10 REPS

The Droopy Mouth Release

Bring softness back to your smile

Mouth corners can pull down due to tension from stress, emotional expression, or facial imbalance. This glide helps release that tension, allowing the mouth to return to a more naturally lifted state.

1 Place your fingers
Place one index finger horizontally across your face, with your fingertip pressing into one corner of your mouth. Rest your thumb on your jawline. Then, place the side of your other index finger gently beneath the first index finger, so that it is resting on the depressor anguli oris muscle (see page 18). You may feel a dip or groove where the muscle attaches.

2 Glide downwards
Glide your lower index finger slowly down towards your jawline, holding the skin taut with the other hand. As you glide, imagine you're lengthening the muscle and undoing the downwards pull it's been holding.

3 Repeat and switch
Practise this downwards glide slowly and deeply 3-5 times on one side, then switch to the other side.

1 MIN

The Chin Smoother

Soften & release tension held in the chin

We usually hold a lot of tension in our chin, which can lead to wrinkles on the chin and mouth area, as well as nasolabial folds. This exercise helps to release some of this tension.

1 **Smooth your chin**
Place your thumbs under your chin, and your index fingers on your chin. Massage your chin deeply and slowly by gliding them down the chin, one at a time. Alternate between each finger and repeat for 1 minute. Keep your jaw relaxed, and allow your lips to part and your lower lip to move around from the motion.

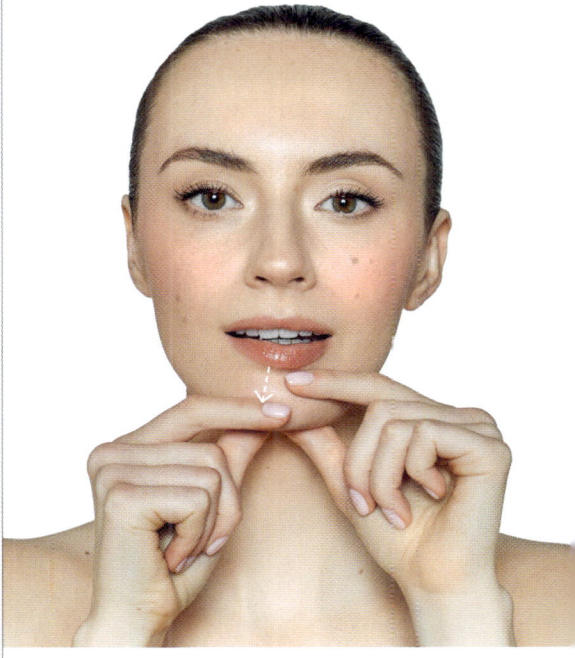

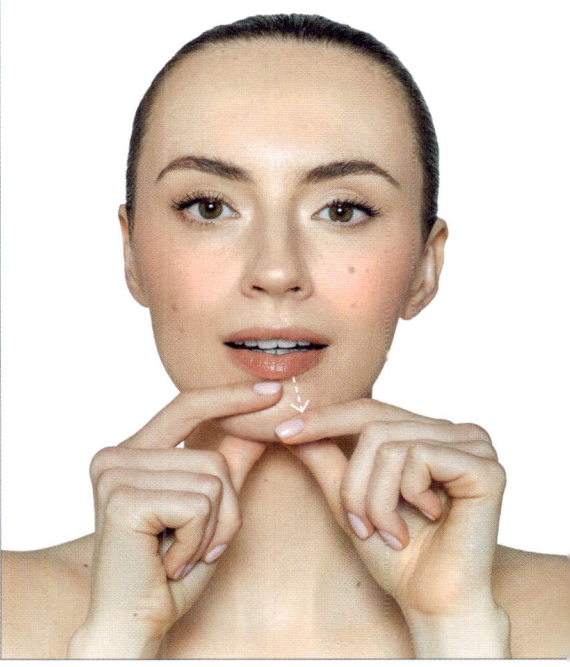

THE METHOD & MOVEMENTS

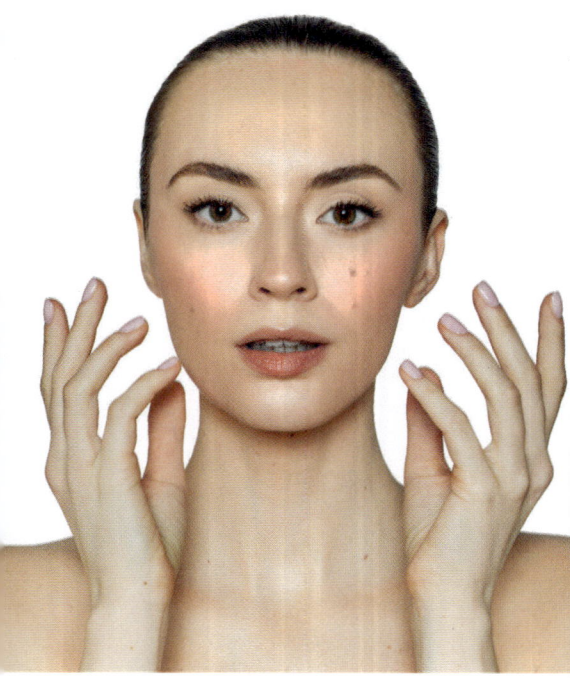

 1 MIN

The Mouth & Jaw Tap

Refresh the lower face & melt away jaw tension

This exercise improves blood circulation in the lower part of your face. It's beneficial for reducing tightness from clenching, softening lines around the mouth, and encouraging a more lifted, balanced appearance.

1 **Tap and pat**
Tap all along the lower part of your face, keeping your fingertips soft and your face relaxed. You can alternate between tapping and patting with the fingers.

2 **Continue**
Continue for 1 minute at your own pace, moving from your mouth and jawline down to the neck, chest and shoulders.

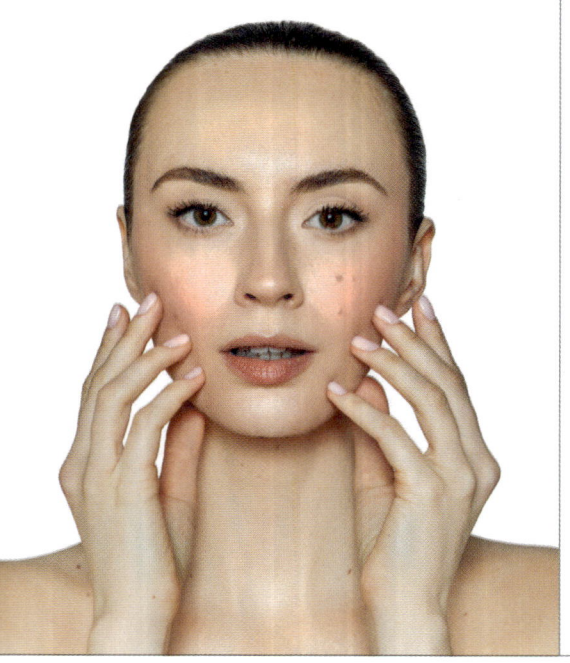

TIP

For the tapping motion, imagine your fingers are tiny raindrops falling onto your skin, or that you're playing your favourite piano melody. For the patting motion, think of gently dusting flour from a surface.

1 MIN

The Jawline Hook

Relieve tightness & support facial drainage

This technique releases muscle tension and stimulates lymphatic flow along the jawline. It's especially helpful for reducing puffiness, softening tightness from clenching or stress, and defining the contours of the face.

1 Hook
Press your thumbs underneath your jawbone and hook your index fingers onto your jawline at the chin. Hold there using firm pressure for 20 seconds, releasing any tension.

2 Move towards the ears
Next, move your "hooks" towards the middle of the jawline, repeating the hold for 20 seconds. Finally, move to the edge of the jawline, almost beneath your ears, and hold for 20 seconds.

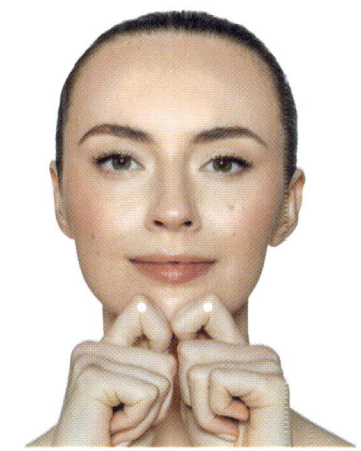
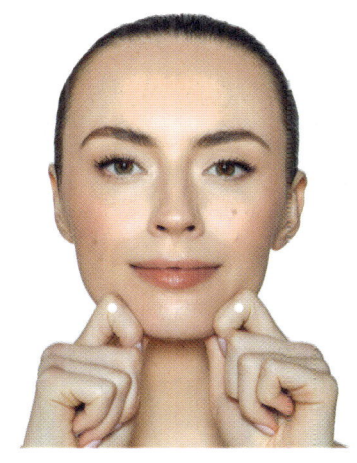
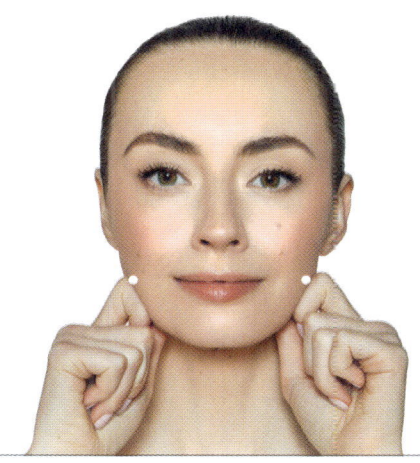

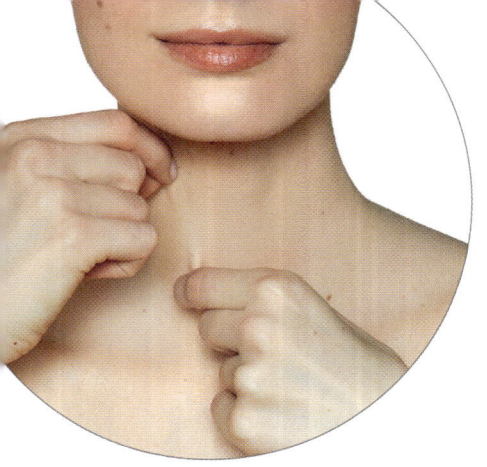

 1.5 MIN

The Neck Pinch

Tone & energize your neck

This exercise improves neck wrinkles and jowels, and prevents a double chin. Don't worry if your skin becomes red during this exercises; this is a sign that you're increasing blood circulation.

1 Pinch the front of the neck
Gently pinch the centre of your neck at the throat, but don't pull on the skin. Continue pinching, moving up towards the chin, and then to the left towards your jaw and ears, and then down the side of the neck. Repeat on the other side at your own pace, so that you are pinching your neck for 30 seconds.

2 Pinch along the jawline
Next, pinch along the jawline, beginning at the centre of the chin and moving towards the left ear and back to the centre. Continue for 15 seconds, then repeat on the other side for 15 seconds, really feeling yourself relieve tension.

3 Pinch the side of the neck
Finally, pinch up and down the side of the neck for 30 seconds, alternating sides.

> **TIP**
> To avoid pulling the skin and to keep your pinches gentle, imagine you are pressing a button between your fingers during this exercise.

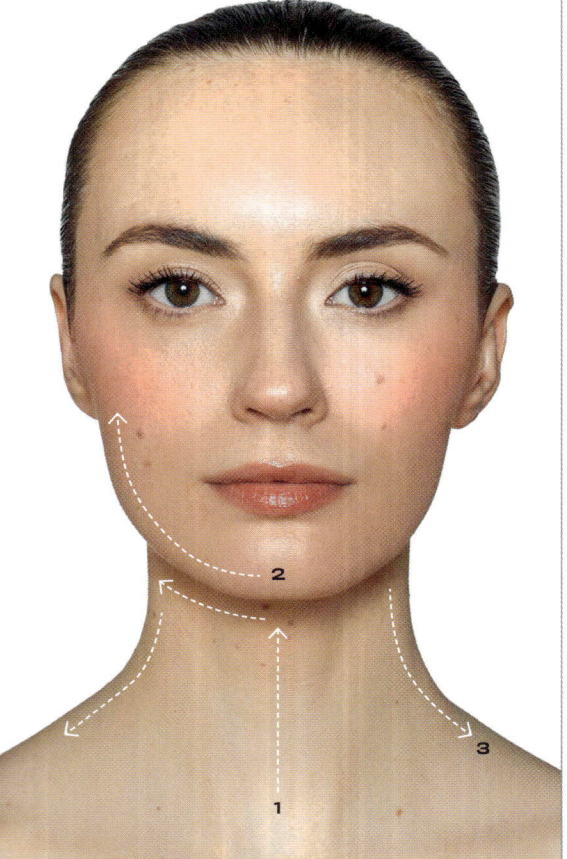

FACE YOGA

1 MIN

The Midi Jaw Sculpter

Depuff & sculpt your jaw

This glide activates the fascia and muscles along your jawline, helping to define the mid-to-lower face. It's perfect as a midday reset or a final sculpting move after release work.

1 Place your knuckles
Place the middle knuckles of your middle fingers so that they are hugging your jawline on either side of your chin.

2 Glide
Glide your knuckles firmly and evenly along your jawline muscle towards the ears, repeating the movement for 1 minute.

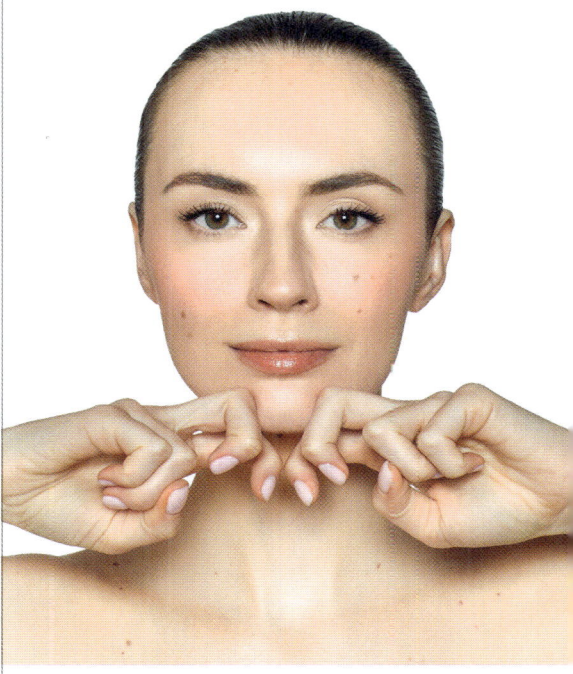
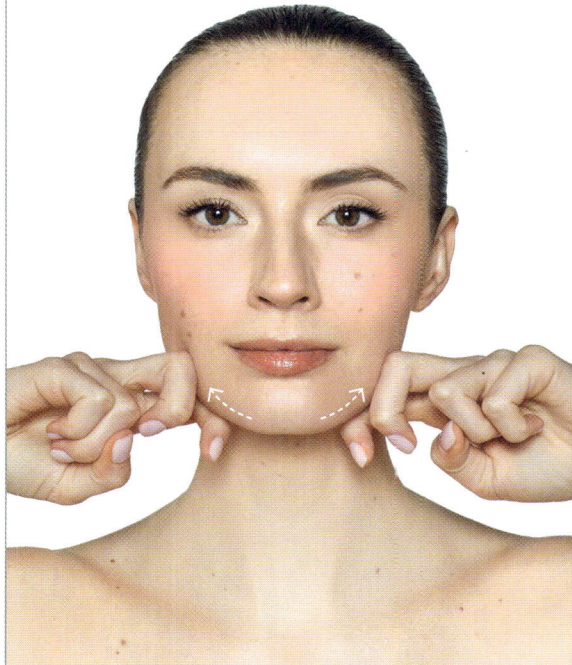

THE METHOD & MOVEMENTS

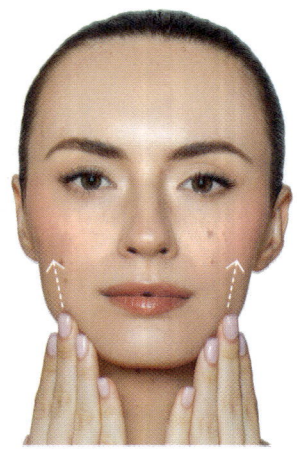

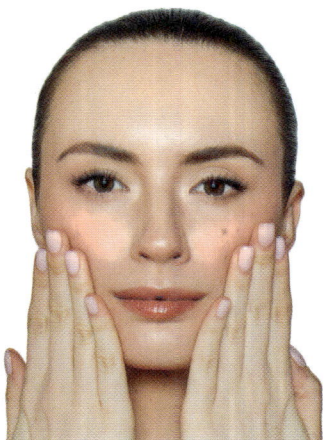

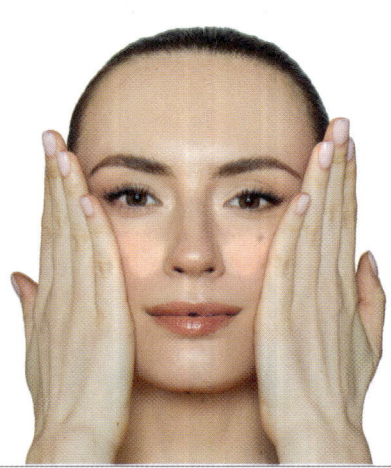

 1 MIN

The Mini Facelift

Give your face an instant lift

This movement releases facial tension while activating the muscles and fascia responsible for facial tone. Over time, it encourages lift, and in the moment, delivers a refreshed, reawakened look. You'll want to use facial oil for this exercise.

1 Place your fingertips
Place your fingertips on either side of your chinbone.

2 Glide
Gently glide your fingertips and palms up and slightly across your face in a slow, smooth diagonal motion, until your palms reach your temples. Keep everything relaxed and use even motions.

3 Repeat
Repeat this movement evenly and slowly for 1 minute, feeling yourself lifting your facial muscles up.

> **TIP**
> *This gliding motion should feel like skiing across snow without any stones in the way. If you ever feel like your hands are tugging on your skin, reapply facial oil.*

1 MIN

The Happy Cool Down

Lift & tone your entire face

This exercise is a great way to relax and set your muscles after any facial exercise or workout. By envisioning how the muscles are lifting and pulling up, it has more to do with your thoughts than it being an active exercise.

1 **Place your hands**
Place your hands on the centre of your face.

2 **Glide**
Glide your fingers up and out with very gentle pressure, envisaging lifting the muscles in your face. Imagine your fingers are light feathers stroking your face.

3 **Repeat**
Repeat for 1 minute at your own pace, keeping your shoulders down and your face relaxed.

> **TIP**
> Think of something that genuinely makes you smile — a happy memory, a person you love, or a little moment of joy. This naturally lifts your mood and activates the muscles that brighten your face.

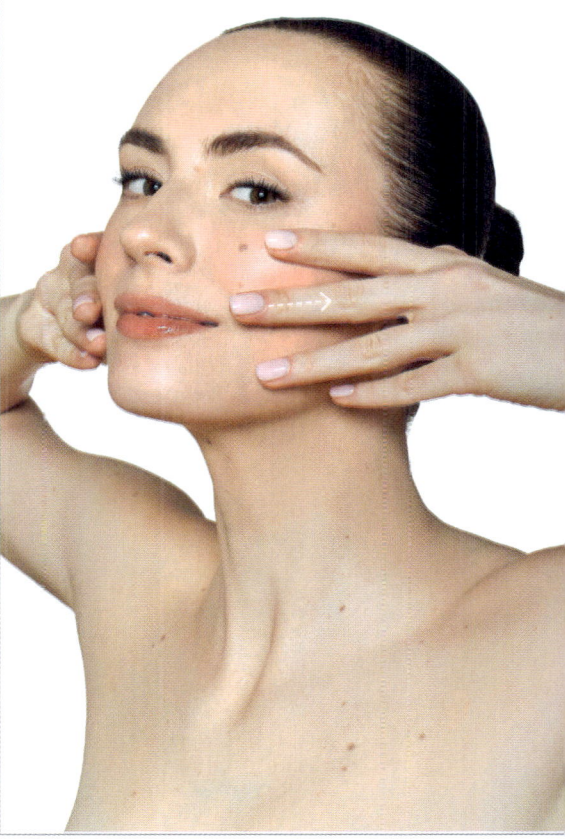

THE METHOD & MOVEMENTS

PHASE 03
STRENGTHEN

Strengthening your face is powerful. It allows you to shape from within, regain natural lift, and gently guide your features into harmony. But it's not about overworking or forcing. These exercises are meant to be done mindfully and in moderation – always balanced with release techniques.

This phase goes beyond simply "lifting" or "sculpting" your face. It's about cultivating a conscious connection with every movement. As you activate and tone the deeper muscles of your face, you'll build not only structure and symmetry, but also awareness – of how you express yourself, how you communicate, and how you show up in the world.

Through this practice, you'll begin to carry new awareness into your daily life, noticing how you hold your mouth when you concentrate, how tension creeps into your brow when you're stressed, and how a softened gaze changes your connection with others.

The Swan Neck 122
The Nodding Smile 123
The Princess Kiss 124
The Cheeky Tongue 125
The Neck Elongator 126
The Double Chin Kill 127
The Giraffe Kiss 128
The Kiss Shaper 129
The Kissing Triangle 130
The Smiling Push Up 131
The Whisper Pose 132
The Tongue Dancer 133
The Symmetrical Smile Line 134
The Blow Up 135
The Roundabout 136
The Cheeky Lift 137
The Nose Shaper 138
The Nose Slimmer 139
The Nose Push Up 140
The Laugh Line & Cheek Lift 141
The Cheek Push & Pull 142

The Spoon Push Up 143
The Smiling "O" 144
The Candle Blower 145
The Cheeky Booster 146
Eye Gymnastics 147
The Under-Eye Push Up 148
The Under-Eye Toner 149
The Under-Eye Lift 150
The Cat Eye Lift 151
The Cat Eye 152
The Eyelid Stretch 153
The Secret Spy 154
The Calm Surprise 155
The Eye Symmetry Workout 156
The Pencil Push Up 157
Forehead Resistance Training 158
The Forehead Finger Push Up 159
The Forehead Smoother 160
The Happy Booster 161

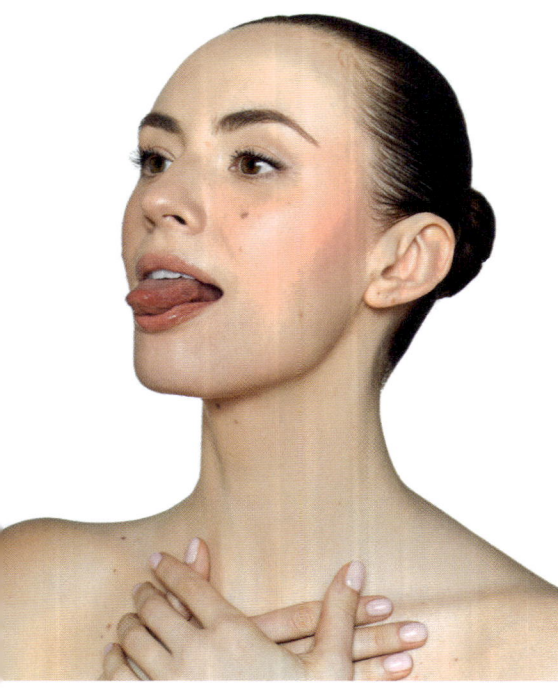
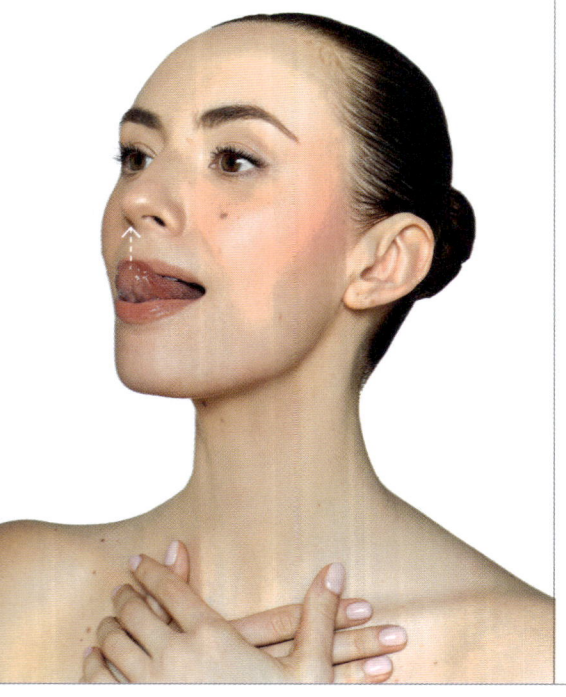

 1 MIN

The Swan Neck

Create elegant length & tone your neck

This exercise strengthens and stretches the neck muscles, helps reduce visible lines, improves jaw support, and prevents the downwards pull that can lead to a double chin or neck creasing.

1 **Place your hands**
Place your hands on top of one another on the lower part of your neck, around your collarbones. This is your anchor.

2 **Look up**
Gently look up to the ceiling. Avoid frowning and keep your face relaxed. Feel the stretch in your neck.

3 **Stick your tongue out**
Stick your tongue out, and then bring it in again. Create a circular motion, sticking your tongue in and out again, as if licking the upper lip, without touching it. Continue for 1 minute.

> **TIP**
> To ensure you're doing the correct movement with your tongue, pretend you are a dog or cat drinking from a water bowl, or that you are licking an ice cream.

1 MIN

The Nodding Smile

Stretch & strengthen your lower face

This gentle yet effective movement helps to firm the lower face and neck. Smiling during the motion also engages the corners of the mouth and supports muscle tone across the jawline.

1 Smile
Smile as much as you can while keeping your mouth closed, and place your hands on your chest. Try to ensure that when you smile, the corners of the mouth are symmetrical to one another, and that you are smiling towards your ears.

2 Nod
Maintaining your smile, gently look up and down, creating a nodding motion.

3 Continue
Continue nodding for 1 minute, avoiding frowning, and keeping your chest open and shoulder relaxed.

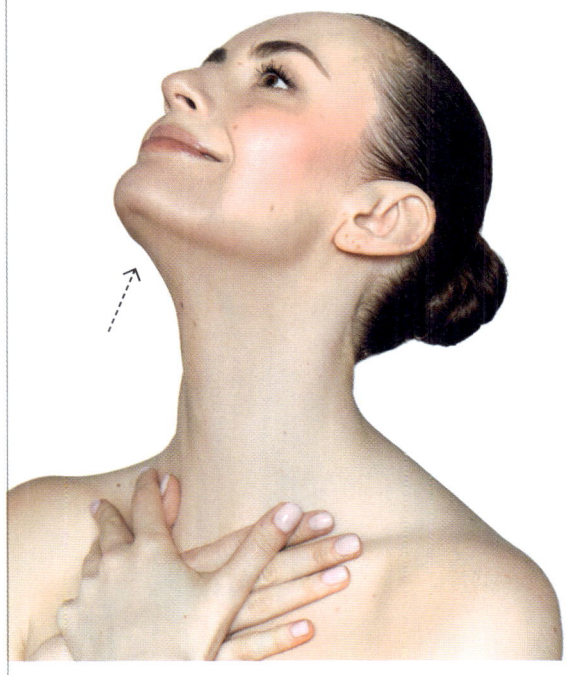

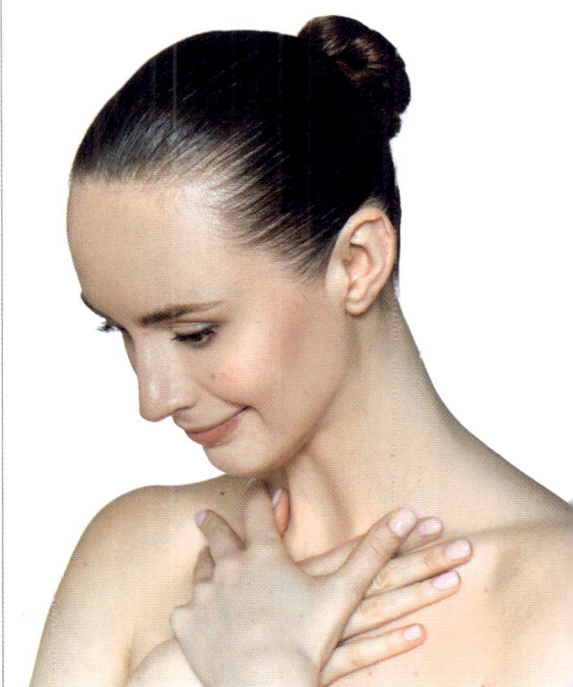

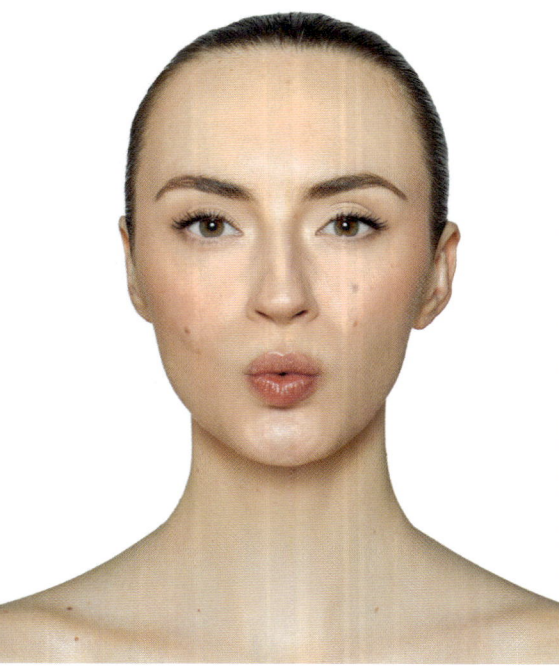

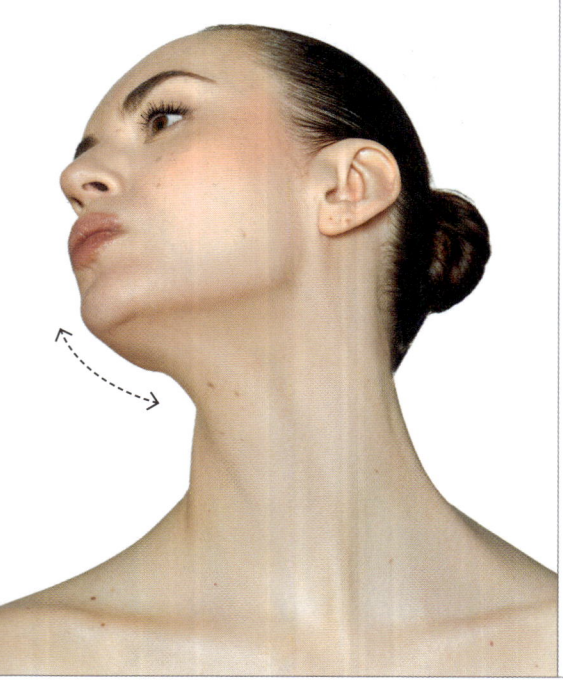

 1 MIN

The Princess Kiss

Tone & stretch your neck

This elegant exercise helps elongate the neck and lower face. It activates the muscles that often lose strength with time, leading to sagging or a "turkey neck" appearance.

1 Kiss
Make a kissing shape with your lips and hold it. Maintain this shape for the full exercise, and avoid creating wrinkles around the mouth.

2 Tilt
Slowly tilt (but don't rotate) your head towards your right shoulder, and then up, as if looking to the right corner of the ceiling. Do this slowly and at your own pace, keeping the kissing shape, and holding to feel the stretch.

3 Repeat
Repeat on both sides equally for 1 minute in total, feeling your neck lengthen and elongate.

1 MIN

The Cheeky Tongue

Release deep tension & tone the neck & jaw

This exercise stretches your neck, improves neck wrinkles and jowels, and prevents a double chin.

1 Place your hands
Place your hands on top of one another on the lower part of your neck – around the clavicle bones. This is your anchor.

2 Look up
Gently look up to the ceiling. Avoid frowning and keep your face relaxed. Feel the stretch in your neck.

3 Stick your tongue out
Stick your tongue out as far as you can, and move the tongue from left to right at your own pace slowly for 30 seconds. Keep your jaw relaxed, and don't forget to breathe. You can keep your eyes open or closed for this exercise.

4 Repeat
Come out of the exercise, take a deep breath, and then repeat for a second set for 30 seconds.

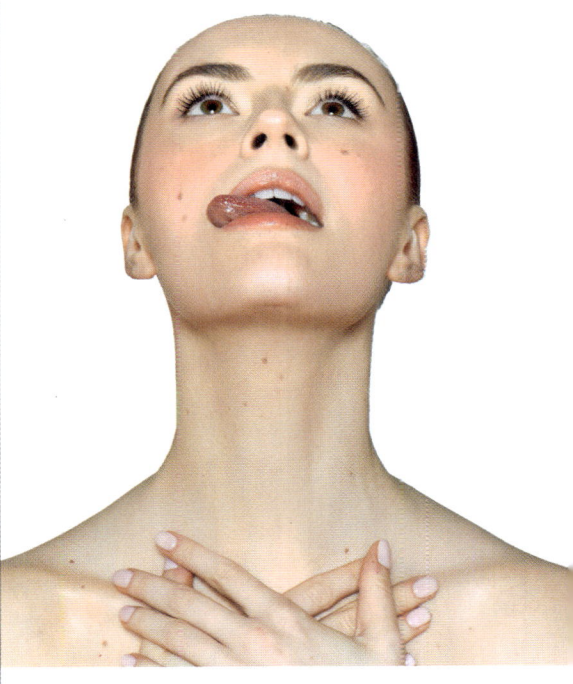

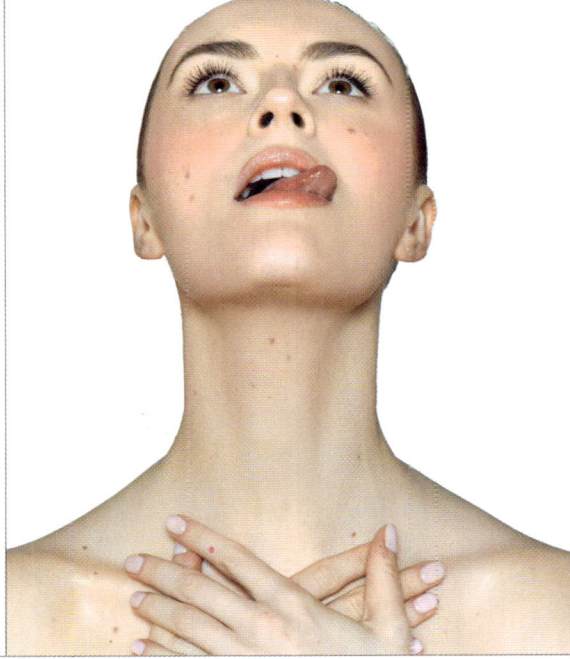

THE METHOD & MOVEMENTS

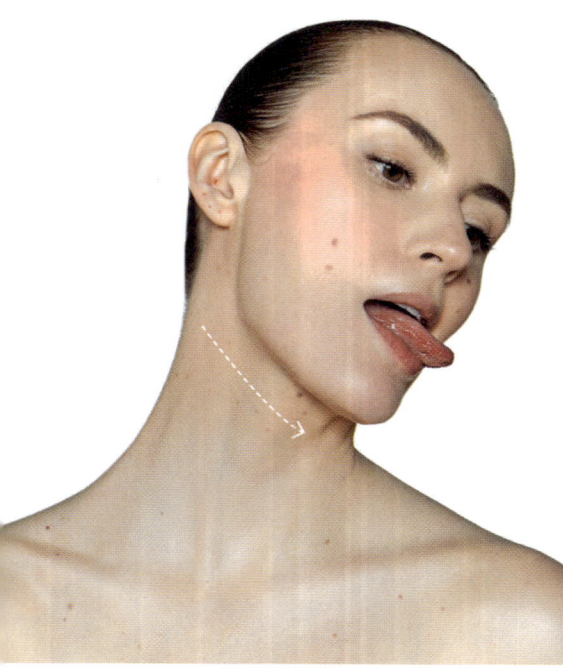

 1 MIN

The Neck Elongator

Stretch, activate, & relax your neck muscles

This exercise uses tongue engagement and directional stretching to activate the deeper neck muscles, release built-up tension, and promote a longer, more graceful neck line over time.

1 **Tilt**
Gently tilt (but don't rotate) your head towards your left shoulder. Feel and enjoy the stretch on the right side of your neck.

2 **Stick your tongue out**
Stick your tongue out to the left side of your mouth. Hold for 30 seconds, feeling the stretch down the left side of your neck.

3 **Repeat**
Repeat on the other side for 30 seconds.

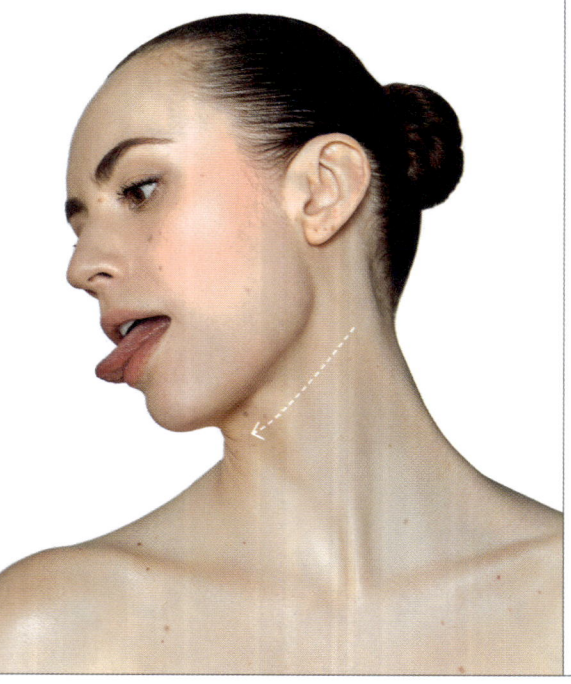

20 REPS

The Double Chin Kill

Strengthen your neck & prevent a double chin

This move targets one of the most common areas of concern: the space beneath the chin. It strengthens the deep neck muscles and helps prevent sagging or softening in the lower face.

1 Place the tongue
Place the tip of your tongue up into the roof of your mouth, keeping your jaw relaxed. Avoid pressing against your teeth.

2 Place the hands
Place one hand flat underneath your jaw, like a shelf, and make a fist with your other hand, placing it underneath the flat hand. This acts as resistance.

3 Press
Press your tongue up into the roof of your mouth, and pulse the tongue repeatedly for 20 repetitions at your own pace to feel the muscles in the chin engaging, gently pressing your fist for resistance.

> **TIP**
> You can do this also without the hands anytime when you are commuting, watching a movie, or in the office.

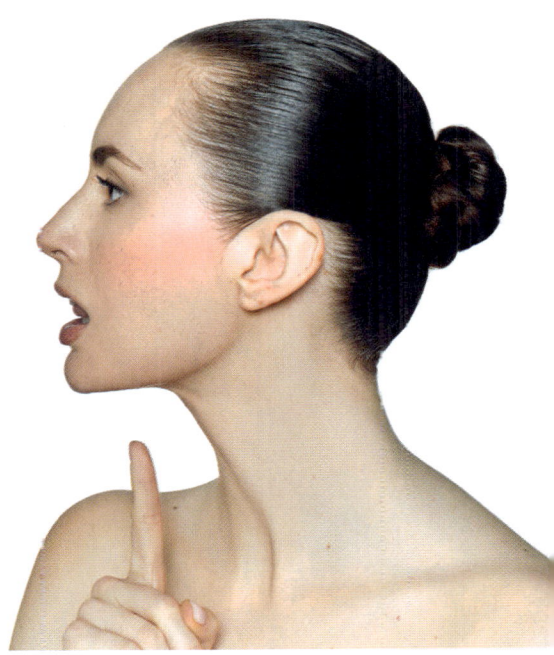

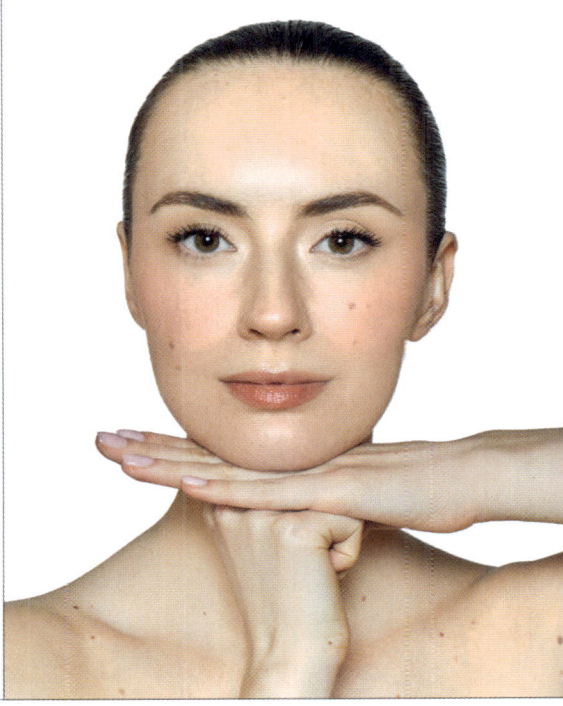

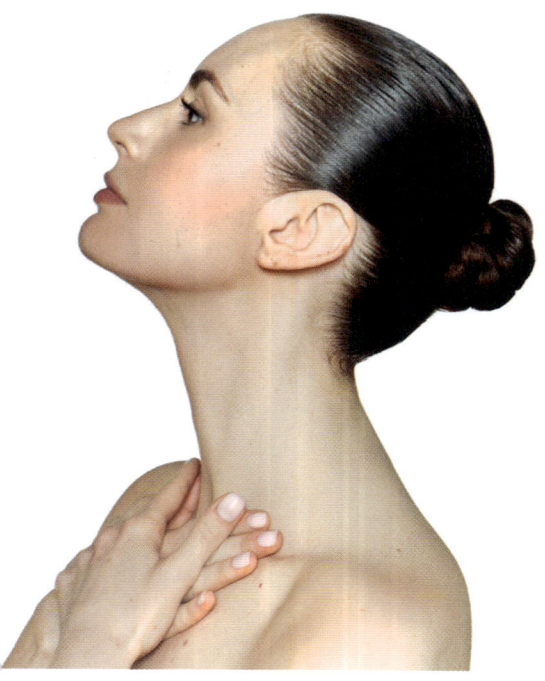
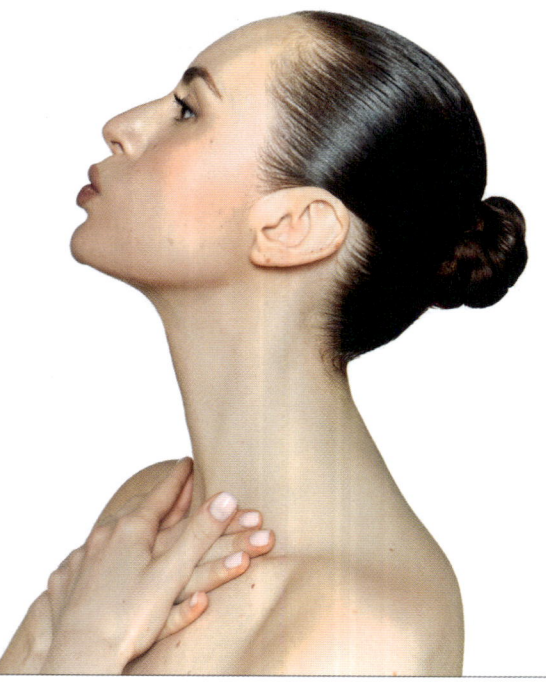

 1 MIN

The Giraffe Kiss

Lengthen your neck & tone your lips

This movement stretches the front of the neck, engages the lips, and tones the muscles around the mouth and jaw. It's especially helpful for counteracting tech neck and lifting the lower face.

1 Place your hands
Place your hands on the bottom of your neck, and look up, feeling the stretch in your neck.

2 Kiss
Slowly blow kisses, imagining you're kissing someone much taller than you.

3 Continue
Continue kissing at your own pace for one minute.

> **TIP**
> *Perform the kiss softly, focusing on elongation rather than intensity. Imagine you're greeting someone from afar.*

1 MIN

The Kiss Shaper

Strengthen your neck & mouth area

This targeted move tones the orbicularis oris – the ring muscle around your mouth. It's a great way to shape and define your lips while supporting overall lower facelift.

1 Place your fingers
Hold around your mouth with index fingers and thumbs. This is your resistance.

2 Blow a kiss
Slowly press your lips out, as if blowing a kiss, and use your fingers to act as resistance against the kissing movement. Relax, and then blow another kiss.

3 Repeat
Repeat this kissing movement for one minute at your own pace, keeping the rest of your face completely relaxed.

TIP
Stay mindful of your breath and avoid over-tensing the lips. The goal is smooth, controlled movement, not force.

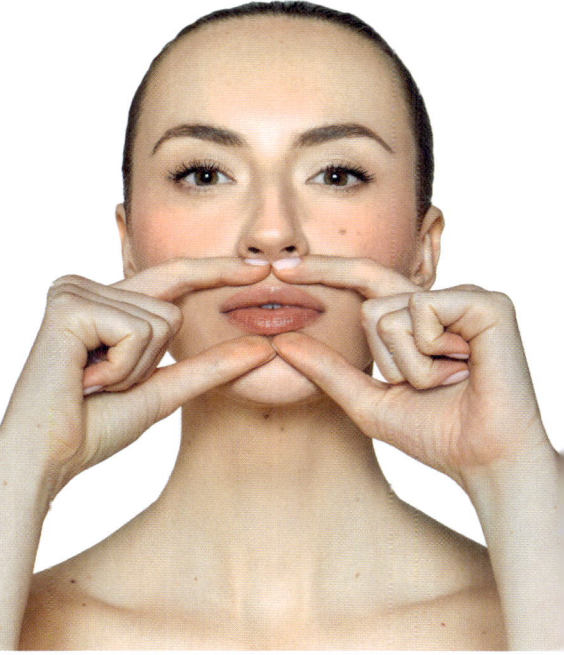

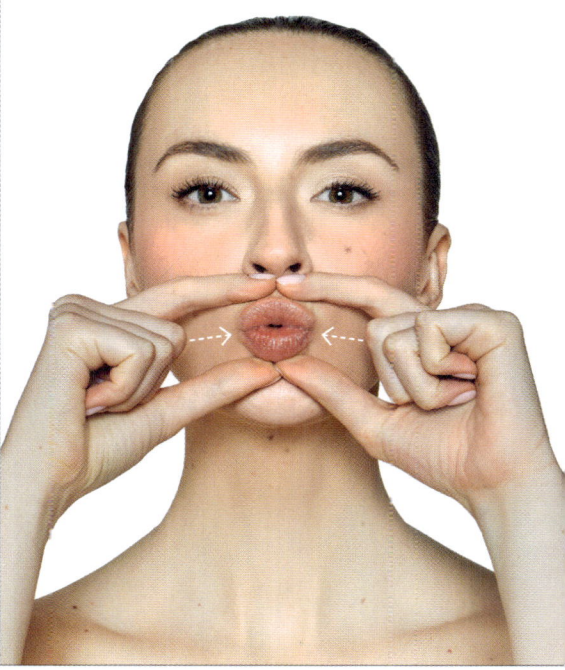

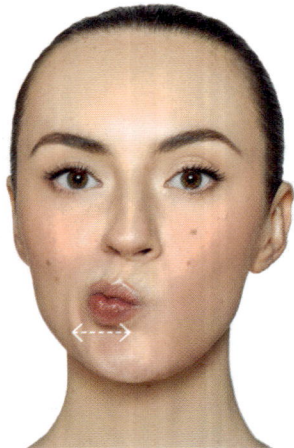
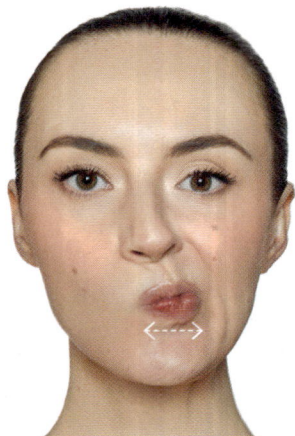
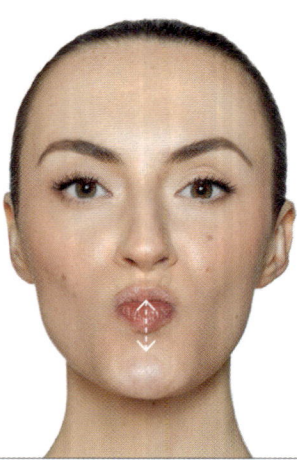

 1 MIN

The Kissing Triangle

Tone the entire mouth area

This movement activates the full ring of muscles around your mouth while enhancing control and symmetry. It brings circulation, tone, and shape to the lips, helping to maintain a lifted, defined look.

1   **Form a kiss**
Place your lips together and pucker them to form a kiss shape.

2   **Create a triangle**
Keeping the kissing shape, move your mouth to the right. Return to the centre, then move your mouth to the left. Return to the centre, and move your lips upwards.

3   **Continue**
Repeat this triangular motion for 30 seconds, then reverse the order, moving from the left, to the right, and then upwards. Switching directions halfway will help improve the symmetry of your lips. Repeat for a further 30 seconds.

1 MIN

The Smiling Push Up

Sculpt & lift your lips

Smiling isn't just a sign of joy; it's also a powerful way to tone the muscles around your mouth. This micro-movement helps sculpt the lips and lift the corners for a naturally fuller, more defined look.

1 **Smile**
Smile as widely as you can with your mouth closed, keeping the corners of your lips symmetrical to one another.

2 **Visualize and lift**
Imagine the corners of your mouth lifting upwards from the inside, as if you're mentally pressing them up towards your cheekbones. You can place your fingers lightly near the corners as a guide, but the real lift comes from within. Keep the rest of your face relaxed and your breath steady.

3 **Hold and deepen**
Maintain this upward intention for 1 minute. Stay focused on the feeling of elevation from the inside. It's a mental push up, not a muscular squeeze.

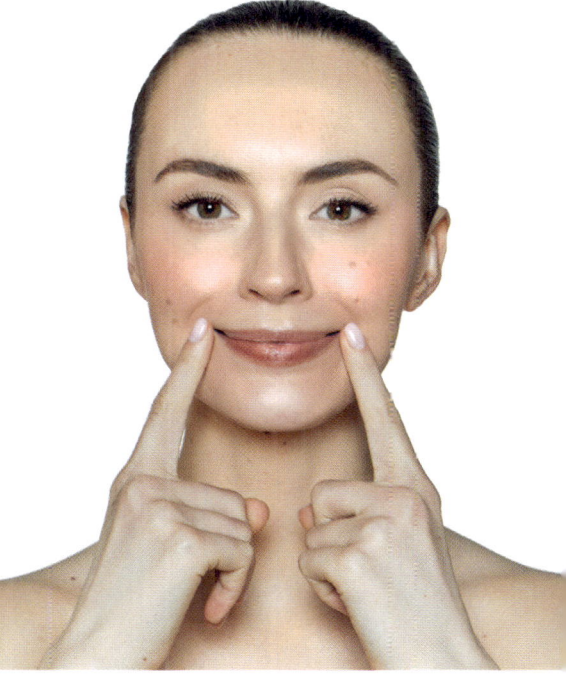

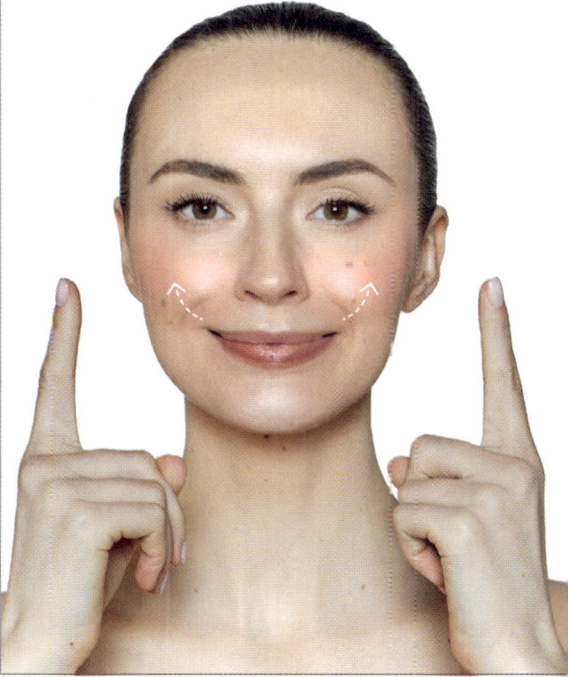

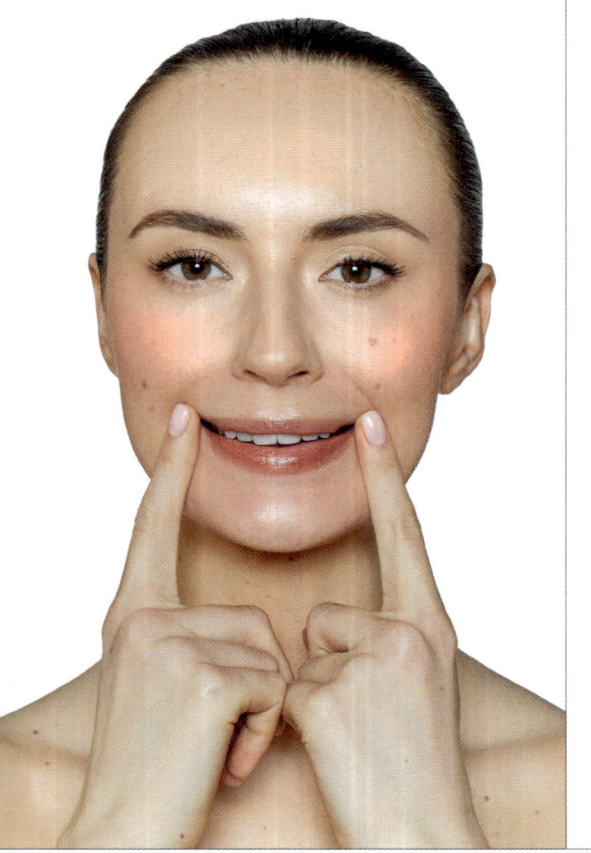

 1 MIN

The Whisper Pose

Awaken your smiling muscles & lift your face

This energizing move tones cheeks, lifts mouth corners, and encourages facial symmetry. It awakens the muscles responsible for smiling and helps retrain the face to stay lifted and expressive.

1. **Smile**
   Smile as widely as you can with your mouth slightly ajar, and place your index fingers at the corners of the mouth to gently lift your smile upwards.

2. **Hiss**
   Holding the smile upwards, say "Ssssssss", as in "snake". The "Sss" sound activates deeper muscle layers while also encouraging calm, controlled breathing.

3. **Repeat**
   Repeat for 1 minute, keeping your smile lifted to feel your mouth and cheeks strengthening.

1 MIN

The Tongue Dancer

Support & improve facial symmetry

The tongue is one of the most powerful and often overlooked muscles in the face. This movement activates the deep facial muscles to support lifted corners and improved facial symmetry.

1 **Smile**
Smile as widely as you can, ensuring both corners of the mouth are lifted equally. You can use your index fingers to help hold the corners of the mouth in the correct place.

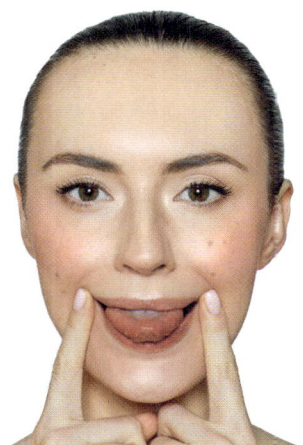

2 **Stick your tongue out**
Stick your tongue out as far as you can, and move it to one side of your mouth, with the tip of the tongue pointing slightly upwards. Hold for a few seconds, before sliding the tongue to the other side of your mouth.

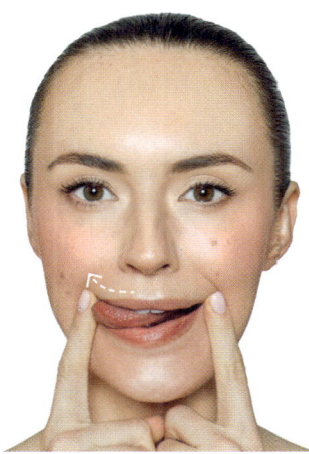

3 **Repeat**
Repeat for 1 minute, moving slowly from left to right in a horizontal line, and feeling the tension in the tongue. Make sure the corners of your mouth stay symmetrical.

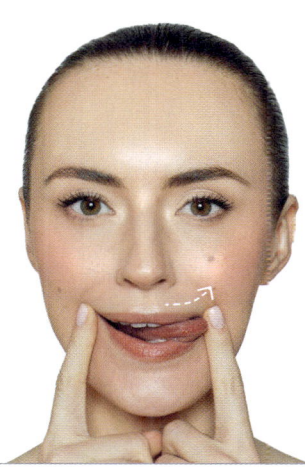

1.5 MIN

The Symmetrical Smile Line

Improve the symmetry of your smile

Our smile is one of the most expressive features we have. This exercise helps retrain your facial muscles to lift evenly, creating a more balanced and harmonious smile.

1 **Grab a pen**
Grab a clean pen, make-up brush or chopstick.

2 **Place the pen**
Place the pen between your teeth in a horizontal line, and cover it with your lips.

3 **Smile and hold**
Smile, keeping the corners of your mouth equally lifted to improve the symmetry of your smile. Hold for 40 seconds, breathing through your nose, and ensuring you're using only your mouth for this exercise, and not the teeth.

4 **Relax and repeat**
Release the pen for 10 seconds and relax your mouth. Then, repeat steps 3–4 for a further 40 seconds.

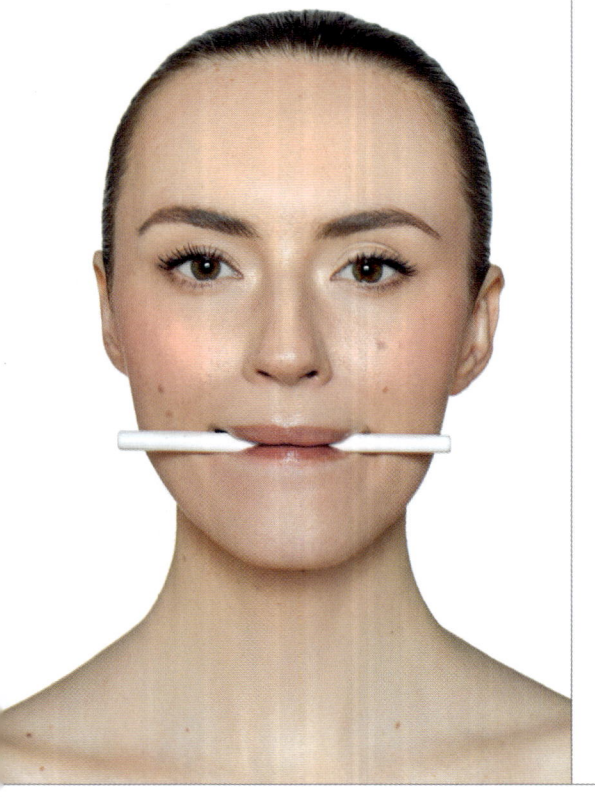

1 MIN

The Blow Up

Strengthen & tone your mid-face from within

This playful movement activates the muscles around your mouth and cheeks, using internal resistance to strengthen and smooth the mid-face. It's a great way to counteract nasolabial folds and encourage facial tone from within.

1 **Blow into your cheeks**
Keeping your mouth closed, blow as much air as you can into your cheeks, filling them up.

2 **Move the air**
Holding the air in your mouth, move the air across to the left cheek, then up to the top lip, then across to the right cheek, and then down to the lower lip. Don't forget to breathe through your nose.

3 **Continue**
Continue moving the air around your mouth in this shape for 30 seconds, then switch directions for 30 seconds, feeling the cheek and mouth muscles working.

> **TIP**
> Imagine you have a little balloon in your mouth, which you are moving from side to side, and up and down.

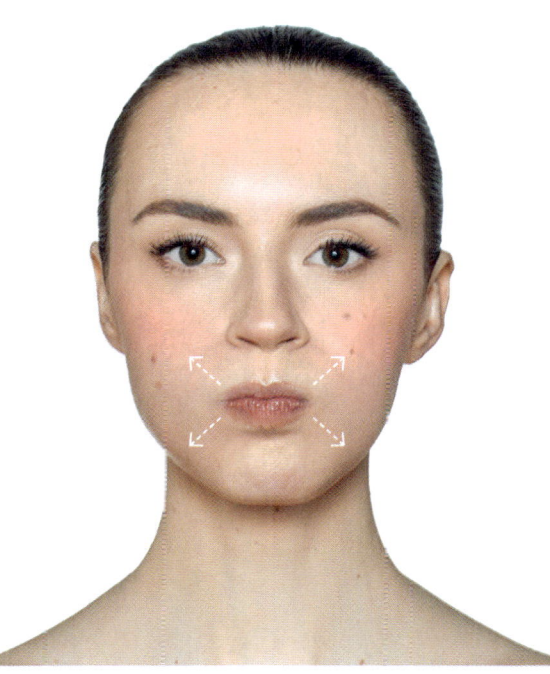

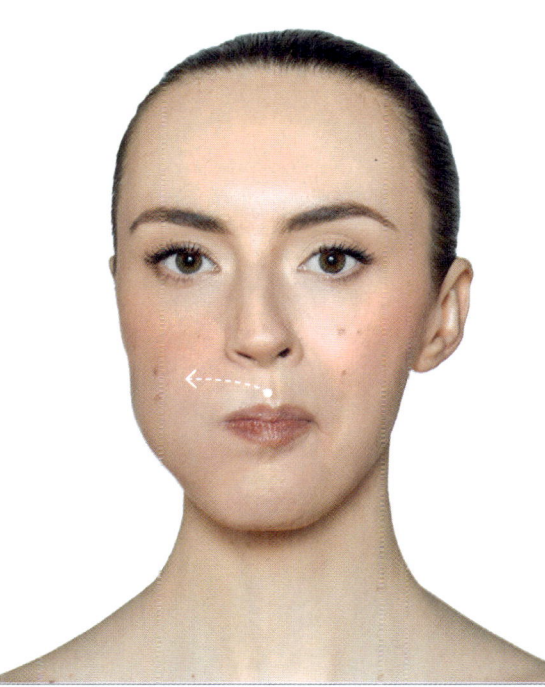

THE METHOD & MOVEMENTS

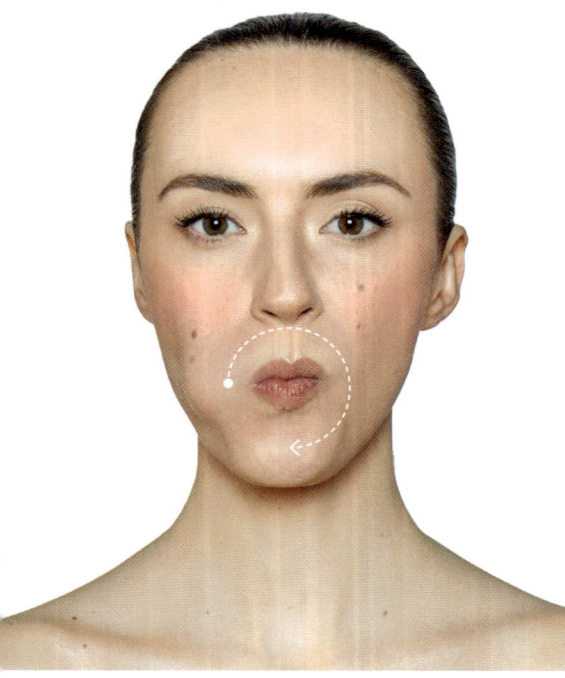
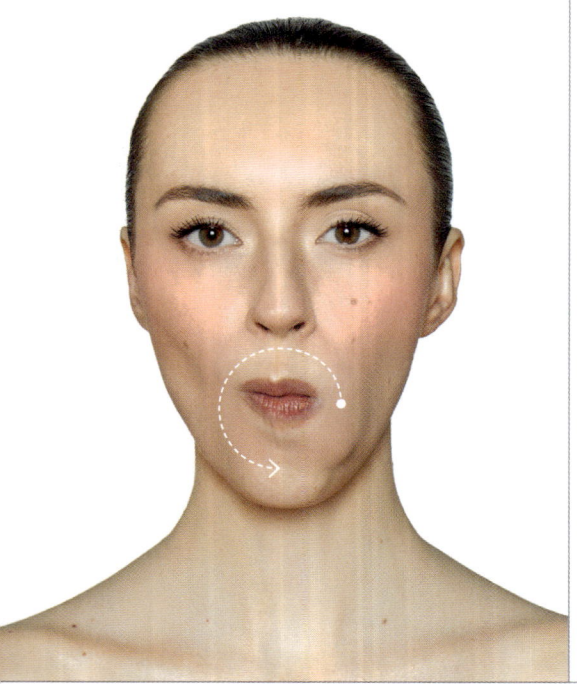

 1.5 MIN

The Roundabout

Sculpt & smooth your cheeks and mouth

This sculpting move targets the deep muscles beneath the cheeks and around the mouth. It helps smooth nasolabial folds and stimulate circulation, all from the inside out.

1 Press your tongue
Close your mouth and push the tip of your tongue up and into one of your nasolabial folds (so your tongue is pressing into the top left or right corner of your mouth, in front of your teeth).

2 Circle
Still pressing into your tongue, move your tongue in a circular motion around your mouth, pressing against the skin of your cheeks and mouth. Continue for 45 seconds in the same direction.

3 Repeat
Repeat, circling in the opposite direction for 45 seconds. Imagine you are ironing out the nasolabial fold from the inside.

1 MIN

The Cheeky Lift

Activate & lift your cheeks

This exercise isolates the cheek muscles to create natural lift and volume. It also helps soften nasolabial folds by training the face to stay lifted from within, rather than pulled expression habits.

1 Cover your teeth
Cover your teeth tightly with your lips and smile, keeping both sides of the mouth symmetrical.

2 Place your hands
Place your hands on either side of your face, and lift the hands slightly upwards to keep the face taut.

3 Hold
Hold this smiling position for 1 minute, using just your cheeks to lift your smile. Keep your shoulders down and your chest open.

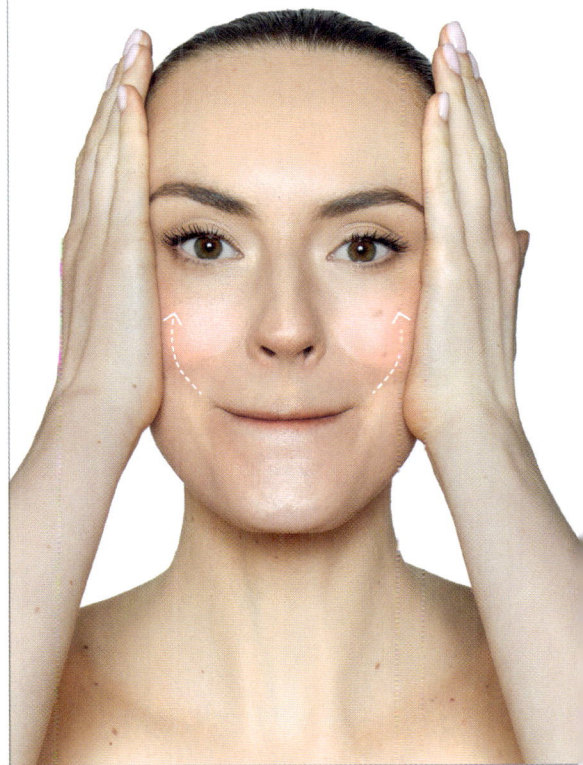

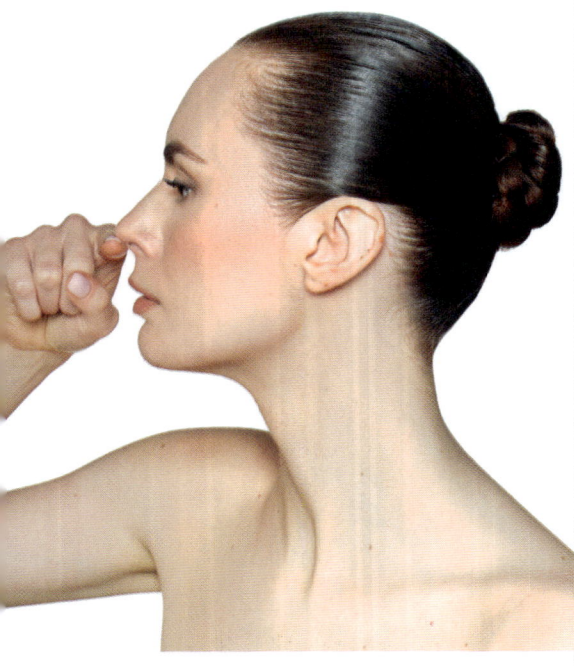
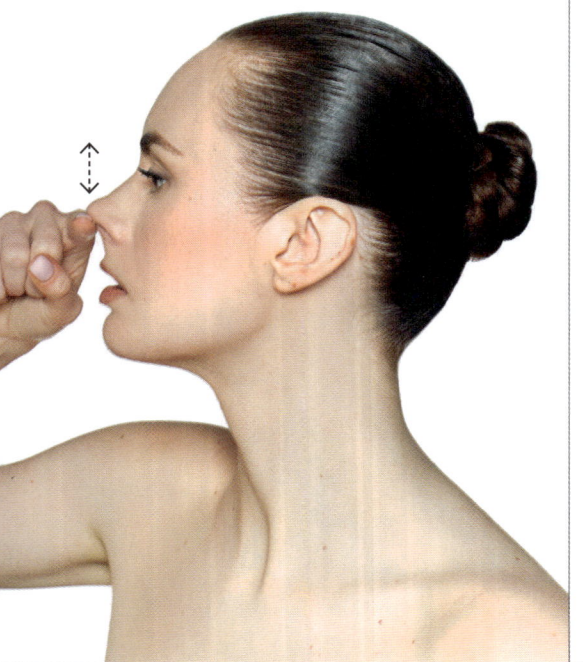

 1 MIN

The Nose Shaper

Strengthen & sculpt your nose

Over time, the muscles that shape the nose can lose strength, causing subtle changes in appearance. This exercise activates these muscles to maintain its defined and sculpted shape.

1 Place your finger
Lightly press the tip of your index finger beneath the tip of your nose.

2 Press
Using just the tip of your nose (not your finger), slowly push your nose tip against the resistance of your finger. This should naturally move the finger downwards. Keep the rest of the muscles in your face still and relaxed, and slightly part your mouth so that your top lip moves with the movement.

3 Continue
Continue this movement for 1 minute.

> **TIP**
> If you find yourself frowning during this exercise, place your other hand gently on your forehead to avoid the muscles from moving, and repeat the exercise more slowly.

1.5 MIN

The Nose Slimmer

Breathe, relax, & sculpt your nose

This breathing exercise engages and tones the small muscles around the nose to help maintain structure, symmetry, and a sculpted appearance. It also encourages mindful breathing.

1 **Cover your nostril**
Place your thumb over one nostril to avoid air from coming through it. Inhale deeply through the other nostril, and hold. The muscles of your nose should start working and engaging.

2 **Switch**
Breathe out, and repeat step 1 on the other side.

3 **Continue**
Continue this movement for 1 minute 30 seconds, slowly alternating between each side, and keep all your muscles relaxed.

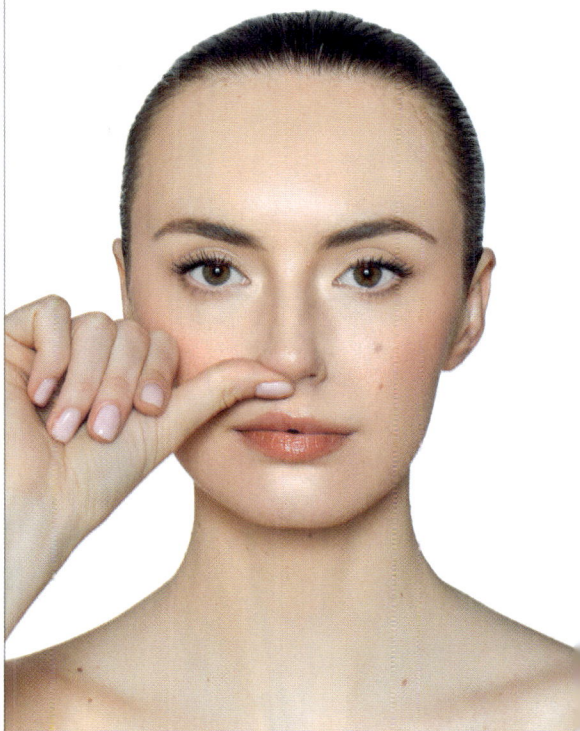

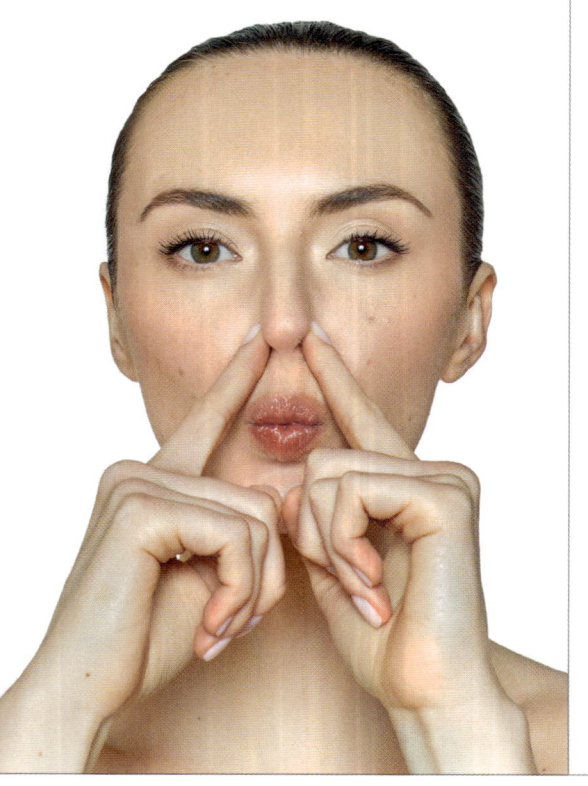

 1 MIN

The Nose Push Up

Maintain a sculpted & beautiful nose

This breathing technique activates the nasalis and surrounding muscles to strengthen the structural support of the nostrils while promoting greater control and awareness of facial movement.

1 Make an "O"
Make an "O" shape with your lips.

2 Place your fingers
Place your index fingers either sides of your nostrils and press into your fingers, so that your nostrils remain only slightly open.

3 Inhale and exhale
Inhale and exhale through the nose, but prevent the nostrils from opening with your fingers. Continue for 1 minute.

1 MIN

The Laugh Line & Cheek Lift

Improve the appearance of laughter lines

This isometric exercise activates the deep cheek muscles while retraining the face to lift from within. It helps smooth nasolabial folds and supports a fuller, more sculpted mid-face appearance.

1 Cover your teeth
Cover your teeth with your lips and smile tightly.

2 Place your fingers
Place your index finger on your nasolabial folds to lift them up and avoid them from forming.

3 Smile
Lift your smile up, using only your cheek muscles. Hold for a second, and then release the smile, but keep your fingers in place. Try to keep your lips wrapped tightly around your teeth.

4 Repeat
Repeat for 1 minute.

TIP
Smile towards your ears and do not engage your eyes.

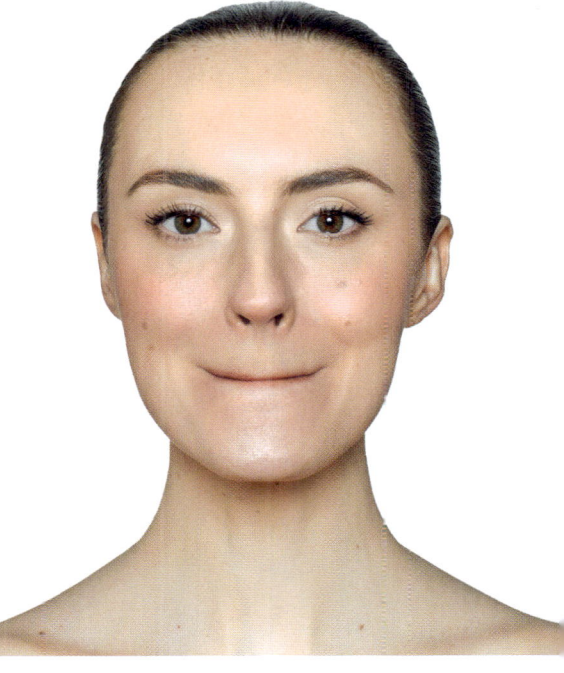

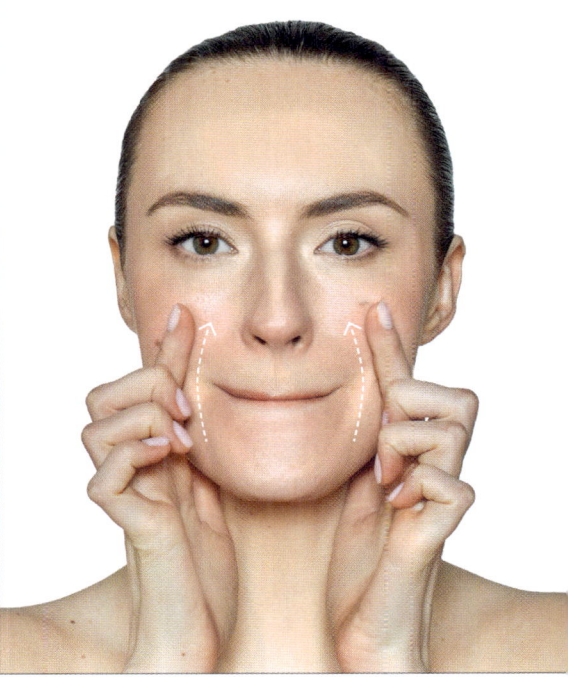

THE METHOD & MOVEMENTS

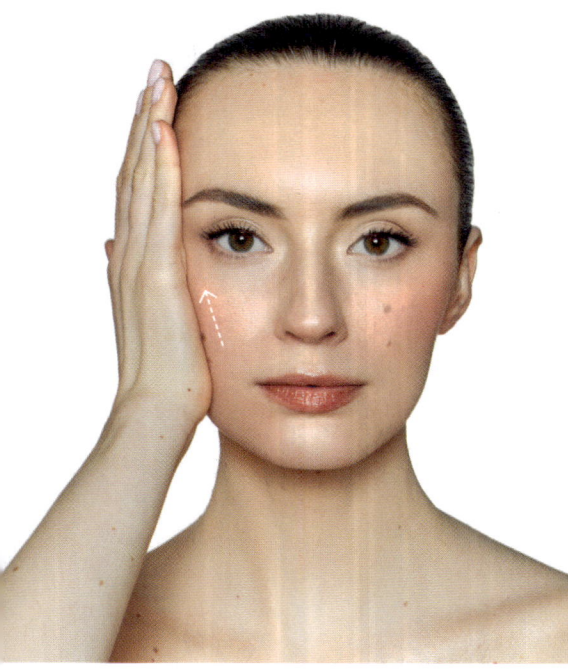

 1 MIN

The Cheek Push & Pull

Strengthen the mouth, cheeks, lips, & jawline

This dynamic movement sculpts the mouth and cheek area by combining resistance with breath. It activates and strengthens the lateral facial muscles while encouraging symmetry and tone.

1   **Place your hand**
Place your right hand on the right side of your face, pushing the hand slightly upwards to smooth out any nasolabial folds, lifting the skin with your hand.

2   **Blow**
Pucker your lips, and, moving your lips to the right, blow air out towards the other side of your face. Actively breathe out through your mouth, and repeat for 30 seconds.

3   **Repeat on the other side**
Repeat for 30 seconds on the other side.

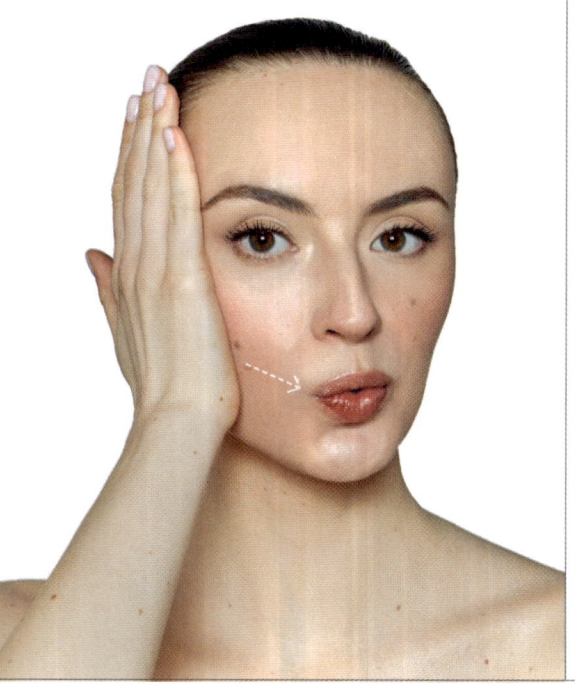

1 MIN

The Spoon Push Up

Tone your cheeks & build a sculpted smile

This exercise uses a spoon as gentle resistance to activate the cheek muscles. By smiling and lifting the spoon, you naturally strengthen your mid-face, helping to define the cheeks and support the smile lines from deep within.

1 Position the lips
Wrap your bottom lip over your bottom teeth, and form a tight straight line with your top lip, avoiding curling it in under the top teeth.

2 Place your spoon and finger
Place the spoon into your mouth. The spoon is there to control the movement. Place your index finger gently on your chin. Your finger is just there to help control the movement, so don't apply too much pressure.

3 Open your mouth
Slowly make the spoon move by activating your cheek muscles – smiling towards your ears. Repeat for 30 seconds, rest, and then repeat again for 30 seconds.

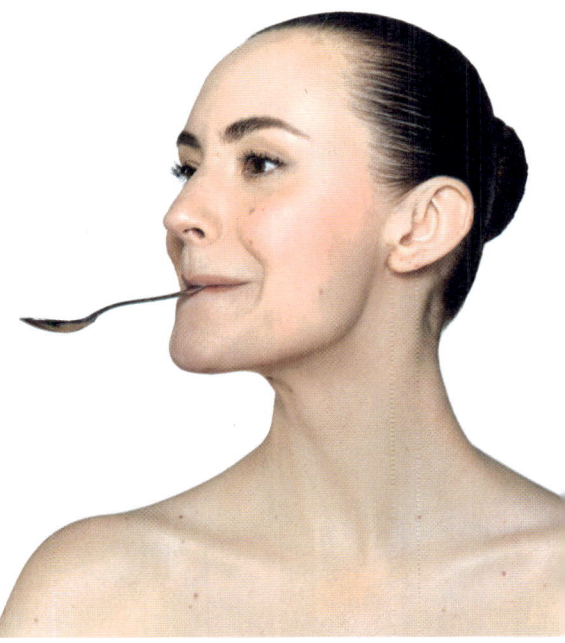
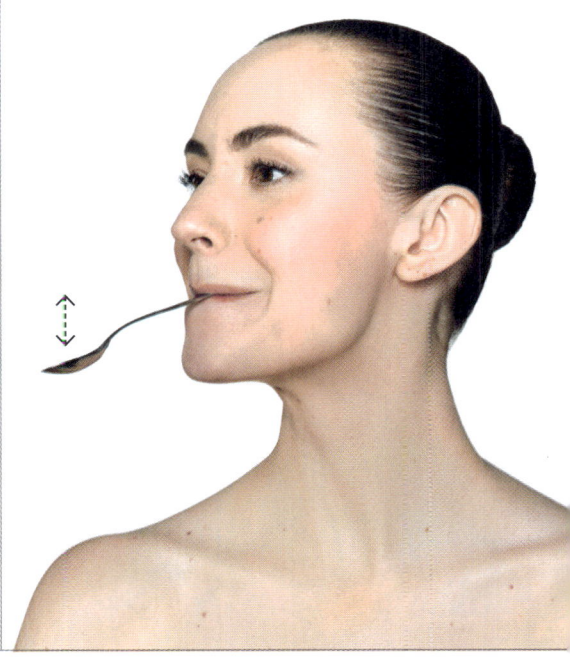

THE METHOD & MOVEMENTS

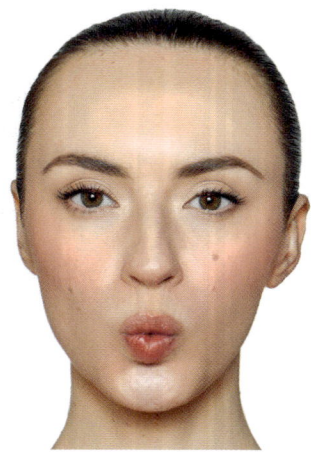
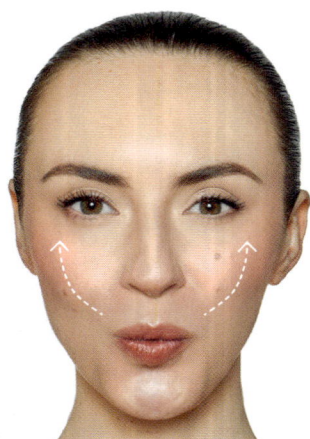
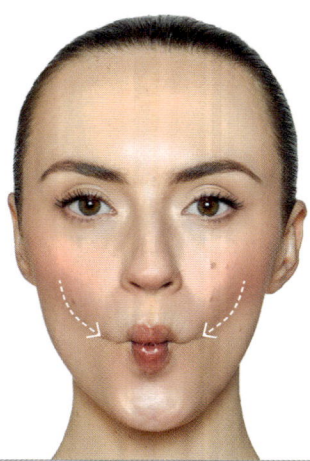

 20-25 REPS

The Smiling "O"

Lift your cheeks & sculpt your cheekbones.

In this exercise, you're activating the zygomatic muscles – the key lifters of your cheekbones. With consistent practice, this movement strengthens the mid-face, supports facial structure, and gives a naturally toned, elevated appearance.

1   **Make an "O" Shape**
Form a sharp, narrow "O" shape with your mouth – the smaller and more defined, the better.

2   **Hold the "O"**
Keep the "O" shape steady throughout the exercise.

3   **Smile Diagonally**
While holding the "O", smile towards your ears using only your cheeks. For more resistance, suck in your cheeks like a fish.

4   **Repeat**
Repeat for 20 to 25 reps. Feel the burn and lift!

TIP
Try to keep your eyes and forehead completely still, as overactivation here can cause fine lines. Focus on isolating your cheeks and visualizing the lift diagonally up towards your ears.

1 MIN

The Candle Blower

Tone your lips & cheeks

This exercise mimics the movement of blowing out a candle. By combining gentle resistance and airflow, it supports firmer cheeks and more defined lips over time.

1 **Place your hands**
Place your hands on either side of your face, and lift the face up slightly.

2 **Make an "O"**
Pucker your lips to create an "O" shape.

3 **Blow**
Blow out slowly, as if blowing out your birthday candles.

4 **Repeat**
Repeat step 3 for 1 minute.

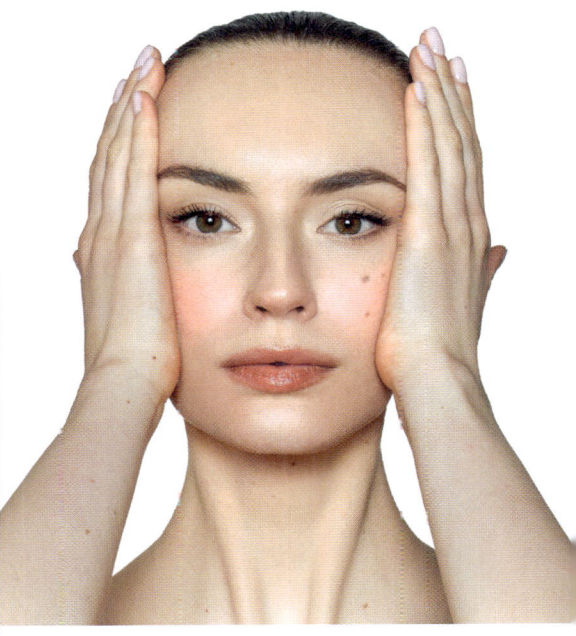

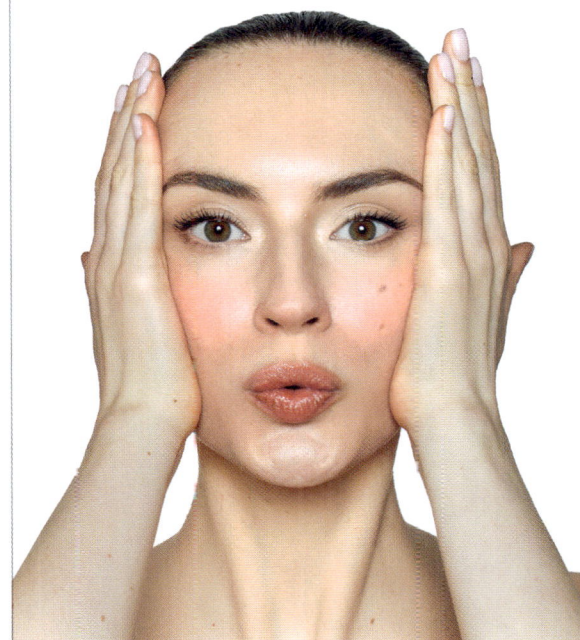

THE METHOD & MOVEMENTS

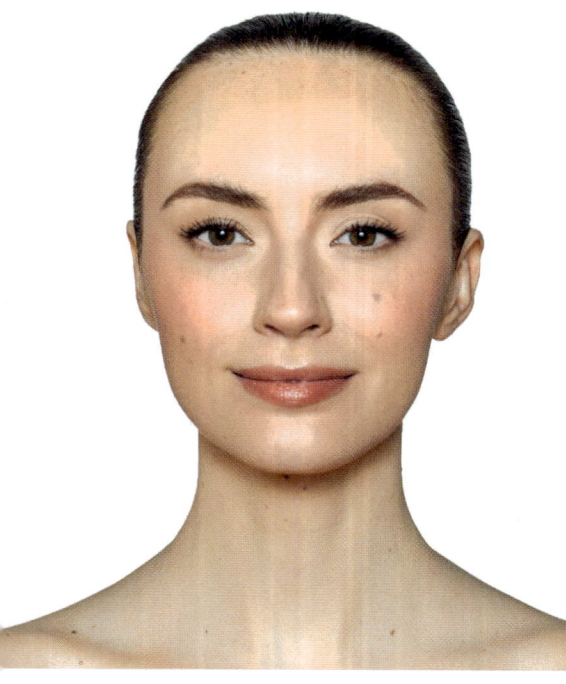
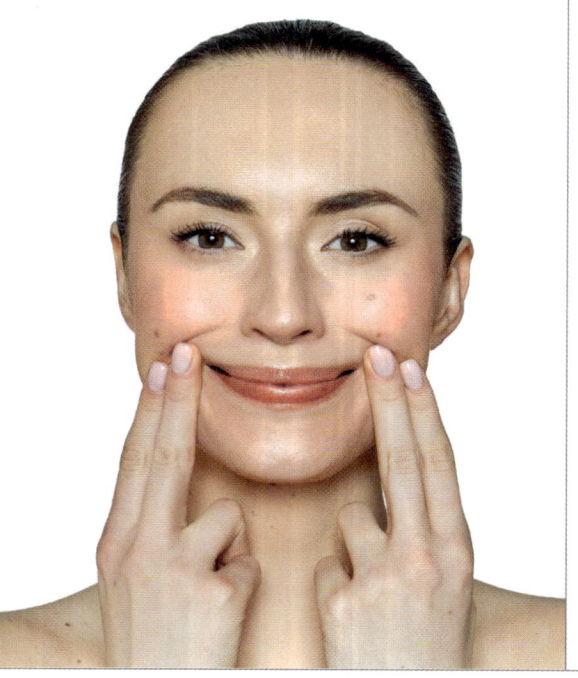

 1 MIN

The Cheeky Booster

Sculpt your cheeks & lift the mouth

This focused movement activates the cheek muscles to promote a lifted, youthful expression and enhance facial symmetry.

1 Smile
Smile with your mouth closed, smiling evenly on both sides.

2 Place your fingers
Place your fingertips on the apples of your cheeks to help smooth out any nasolabial folds.

3 Hold
Hold the smile for 1 minute, engaging the muscles in the apples of your cheeks only, and maintaining the intensity of the smile without frowning or tensing your shoulders.

> **TIP**
> Smile towards your ears, and make sure not to engage your eyes. Keep the effort in your cheeks only.

FACE YOGA

1.5 MIN

Eye Gymnastics

Wake up & activate your eye muscles

This gentle movement sequence activates the full range of the eye muscles, boosting circulation, reducing strain, and refreshing tired eyes. It's like a wake-up workout for your vision and expression.

1 Look to the side
Keeping your head still and facing forwards, look from left to right for 30 seconds. Have something to focus on in each corner to keep this movement controlled.

2 Look up and down
Look up and down for 30 seconds.

3 Look around
Look around, creating an even-sized circle with your eyes. Repeat for 15 seconds in one direction, and then repeat in the opposite direction for 15 seconds.

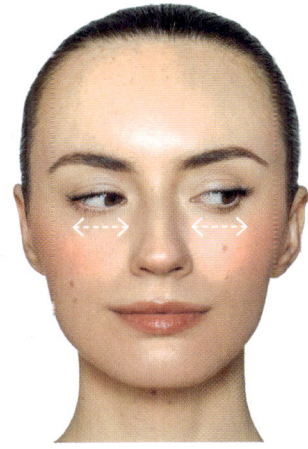
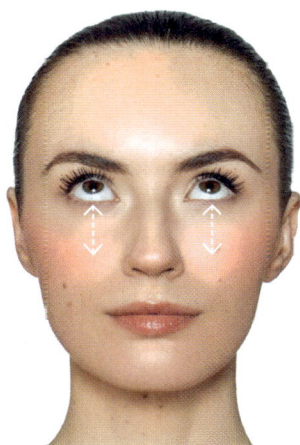
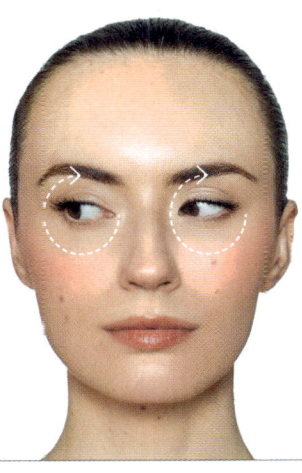

THE METHOD & MOVEMENTS

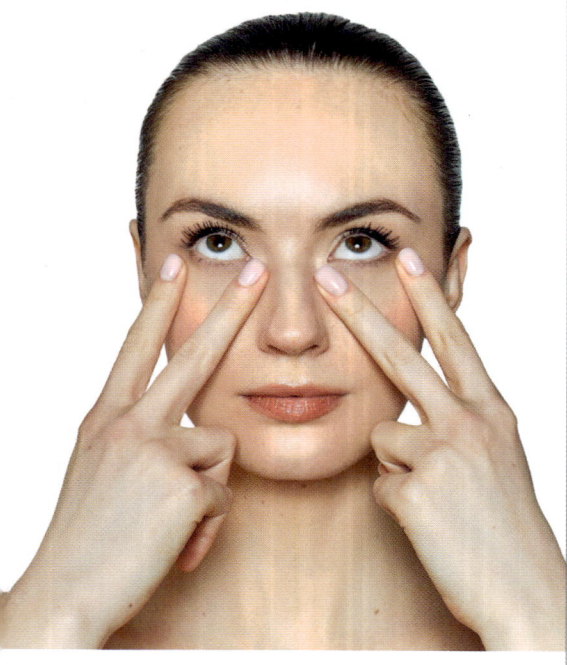

 1 MIN

The Under-Eye Push Up

Plump & tone your under-eyes

This isolated, targeted move helps to reduce puffiness, smooth fine lines, and strengthen the under-eye area without creating tension in other parts of the face.

1 Place your fingers
Using light pressure, place your index and middle fingers on the inner and outer corners of your eyes for resistance.

2 Look up
Look up, and try to squint your eyes by engaging just your under-eyes. Hold for a second, and then relax.

3 Repeat
Repeat this under-eye push up motion for 1 minute. If your muscles start to tremble, this is a good sign.

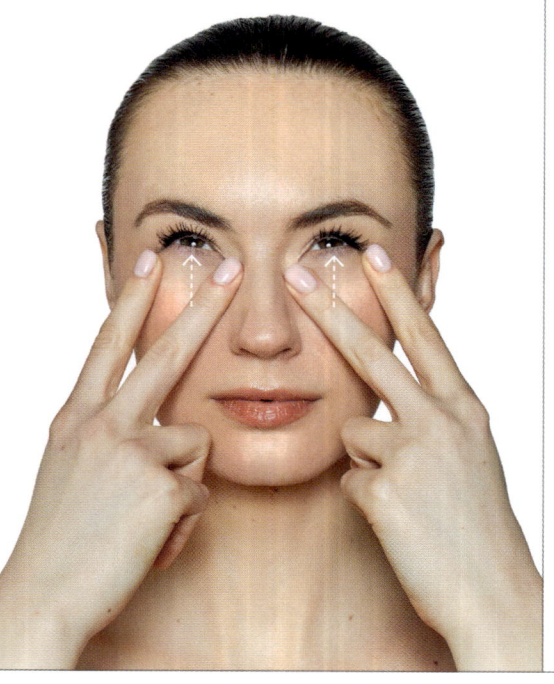

TIP

If your feel your forehead muscles engaging and wrinkling, practise the movement at a slower pace, or engage the eyes less intensely.

1 MIN

The Under-Eye Toner

Strengthen underused under-eye muscles

This exercise targets the lower part of the eye ring muscle to gently tone and awaken the under-eye area without over-engaging the forehead.

1 Place your hands
Place your hands on your temples and slightly lift your face.

2 Look up
Look up, and squint your under-eyes as tightly as you can. Avoid frowning your forehead, and relax all other facial muscles.

3 Hold
Hold for 1 minute.

TIP
Focus on the muscle under the eyes, not the eyelids or brows. If your forehead starts to wrinkle, ease the intensity and try again with more control.

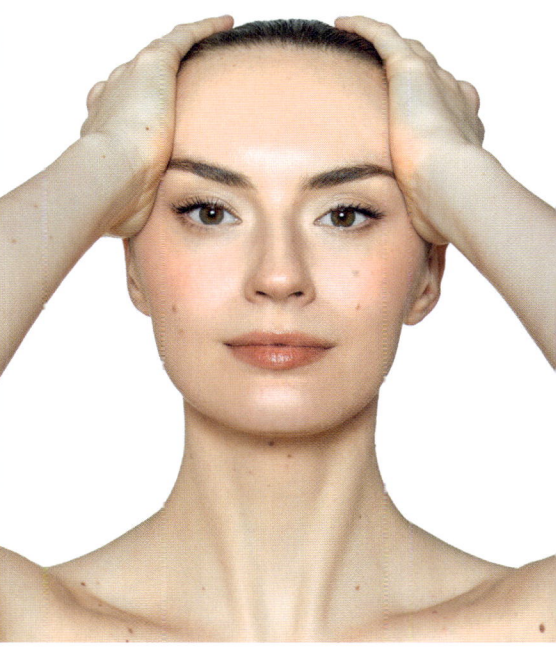

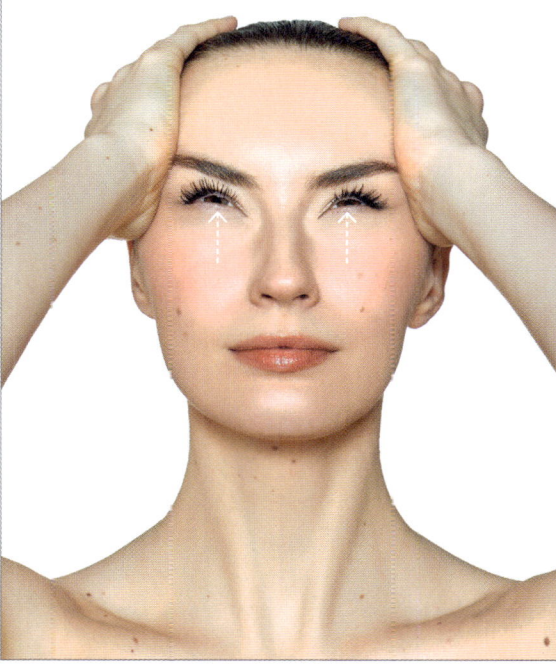

THE METHOD & MOVEMENTS

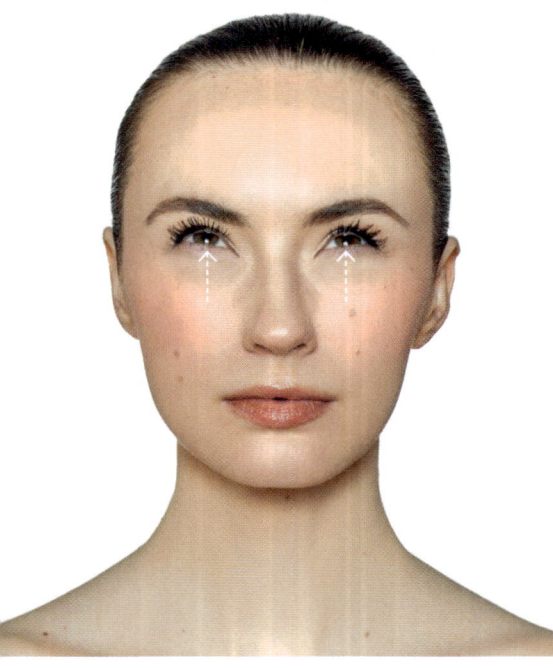

 1.1 MIN

The Under-Eye Lift

Depuff & rejuvenate under-eyes

The under-eye area can quickly show signs of fatigue, stress, or poor circulation. This targeted movement reduces puffiness, tones the skin, and awakens tired eyes.

1 **Look up and squint**
Look up, and squint, trying to use just your under-eyes to lift the lower eyelid. Do not raise your eyebrows, and keep your forehead smooth.

2 **Place your fingers**
Holding the squint, place your index fingers gently beneath your under-eyes. Do not apply pressure; they are just there to indicate where you should be feeling the resistance. If you feel them slightly trembling, that's a sign that they are working.

3 **Hold and repeat**
Hold for 30 seconds, and then relax for 10 seconds. Repeat for a second round of 30 seconds.

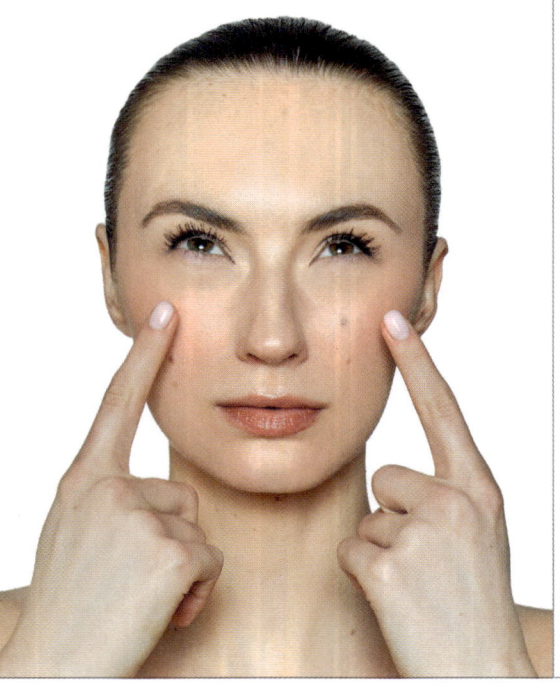

1 MIN

The Cat Eye Lift

Instantly stretch & lift your eyes

This exercise helps lift the outer corners of your eyes, relax facial tension, and refresh a tired gaze. It also helps train upwards muscle engagement and supports a more open, elongated eye shape.

1 Place your hands
Place your palms on either side of your eyebrows.

2 Create the lift
Gently pull your hands upwards and outwards to feel a stretch around your outer-eye area.

3 Blink
While holding the stretch, slowly look down and blink, keeping your head still. Keep blinking for 1 minute, and don't lose tension with your hands. Feel the stretch while all the other muscles in your face remain relaxed.

> **TIP**
> Avoid wrinkling your forehead while lifting the corners of your eyebrows gently.

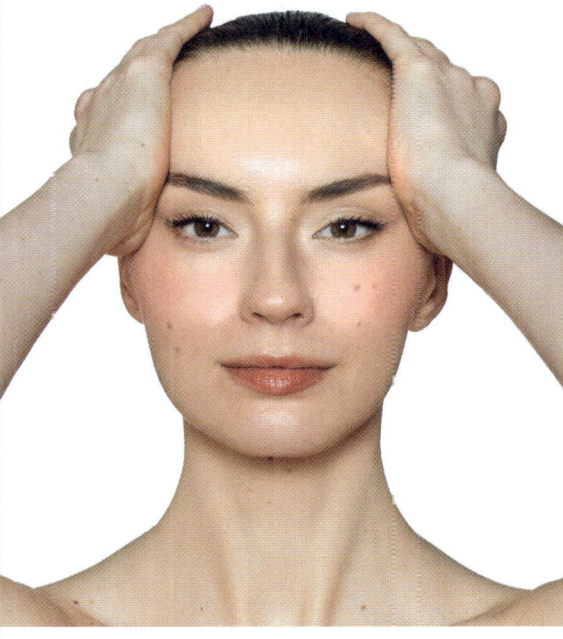
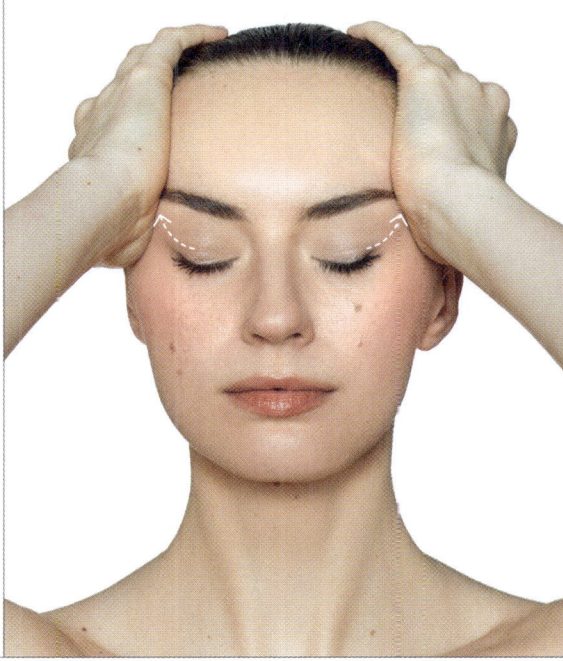

THE METHOD & MOVEMENTS

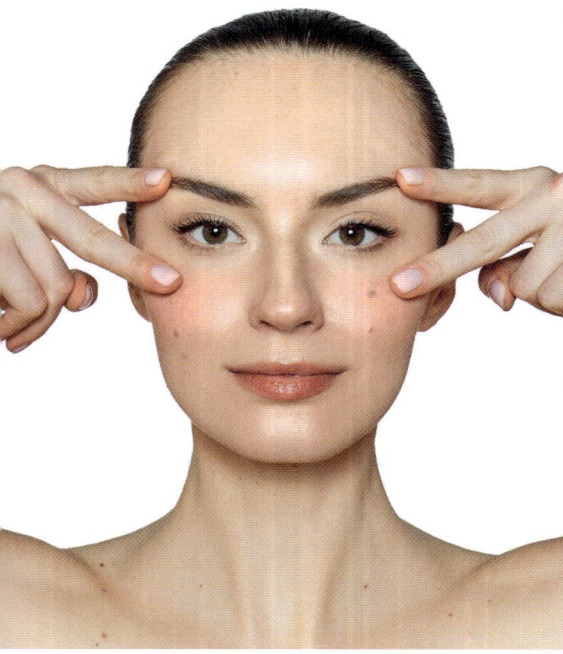
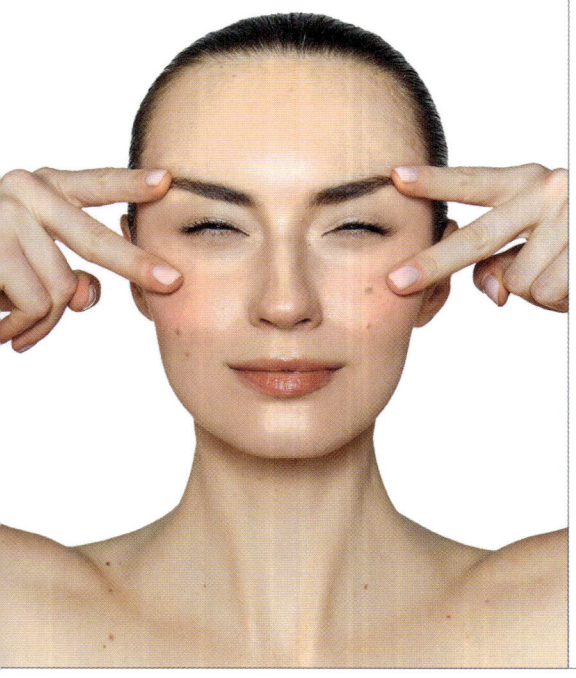

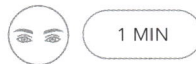 1 MIN

The Cat Eye

Lift & tone your eye area

This exercise targets the outer corners of your eyes, which is often one of the first areas to show signs of tiredness or sagging. By gently squinting, you improve tone for a refreshed look.

1 **Place your fingers**
Place your middle and index fingers on either side of your eyes, with your index finger resting at the outer edge of your eyebrow, and your middle finger resting directly below it beneath the under-eye. Gently press into the fingers and lift them up and out to tauten the skin around the eyes.

2 **Squint**
Squint your eyes, as if you were looking at the sun, and feel the gentle resistance of your fingers. Squint for just a second, and then relax.

3 **Repeat**
Repeat this squinting movement for one minute, letting the eye muscles do the work, and keeping the tension in the fingers to act as resistance.

1 MIN

The Eyelid Stretch

Depuff & relax your upper eyes

This stretch targets the upper eyelids, helping to release tension, reduce puffiness, and restore openness. It's especially beneficial after long periods of screen time or tiredness.

1 Place your palms
Place your palms on your forehead, just above your eyebrows. Lightly pull your forehead upwards, making sure you're pulling the muscle, not the skin.

2 Look down
Look down, and slowly blink.

3 Repeat
Repeat step 2 for 1 minute, feeling the stretch in your upper eyelids.

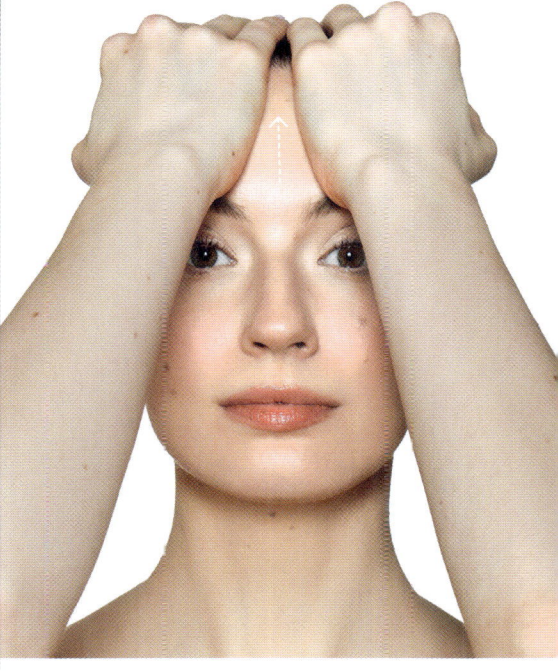

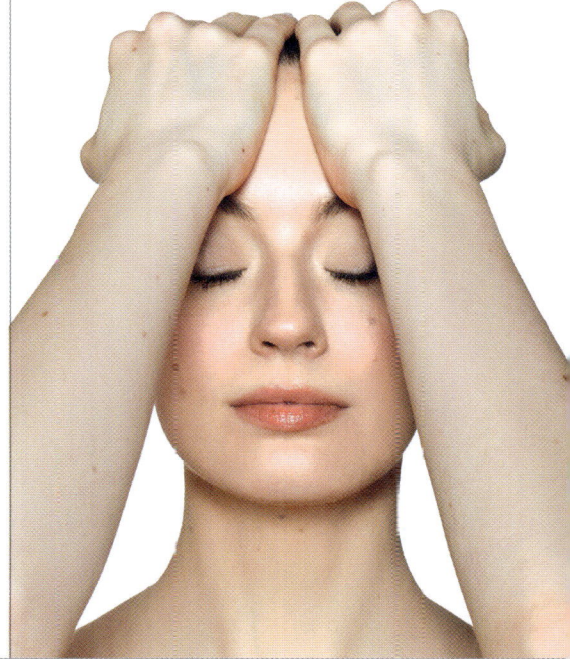

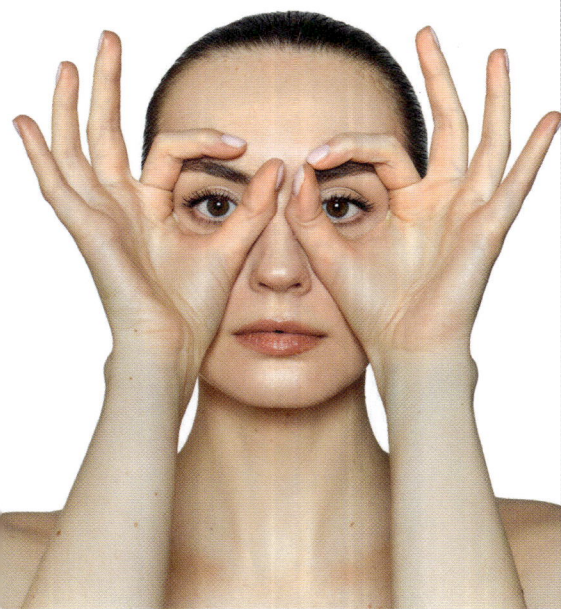
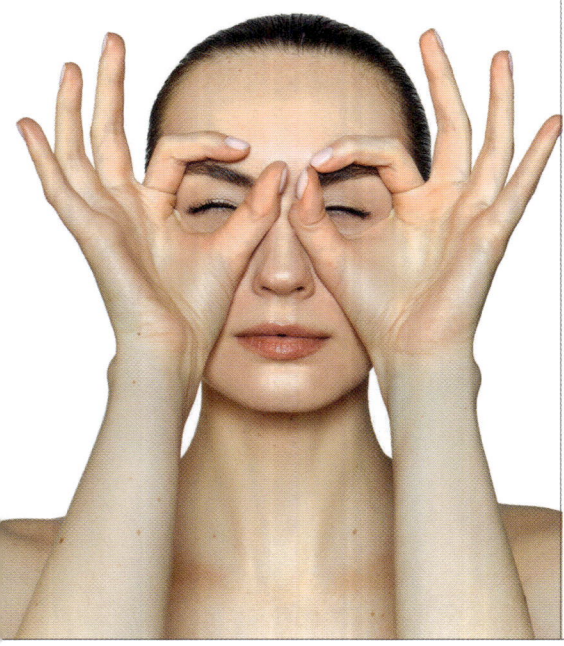

 1 MIN

The Secret Spy

Strengthen your eyes & smooth your forehead

This exercise helps train and strengthen the ring muscle around your eyes, which is responsible for blinking, squinting, and supporting the shape of the eyes.

1 Place your fingers
Place your thumbs and index fingers in a circle around your eyes, imagining that you're looking through two spyglasses. You want your fingers and inner side of your hands to be making contact with your skin at all points, so adjust your hands if any part of your hand is not touching your face.

2 Squint
With your hands placed around your eyes, squint your eyes for a second. Then release them. Repeat this five times against the resistance of your fingers.

3 Widen your eyes
Once you've squinted five times, open your eyes as widely as you can, and hold for a few seconds.

4 Repeat
Repeat steps 2 and 3, alternating between the two, for 1 minute. Avoid frowning and keep your face relaxed.

1 MIN

The Calm Surprise

Activate & strengthen your facial awareness

This exercise helps build facial awareness and expression control without activating the forehead. Over time, this strengthens the eye muscles while keeping your forehead smooth and relaxed.

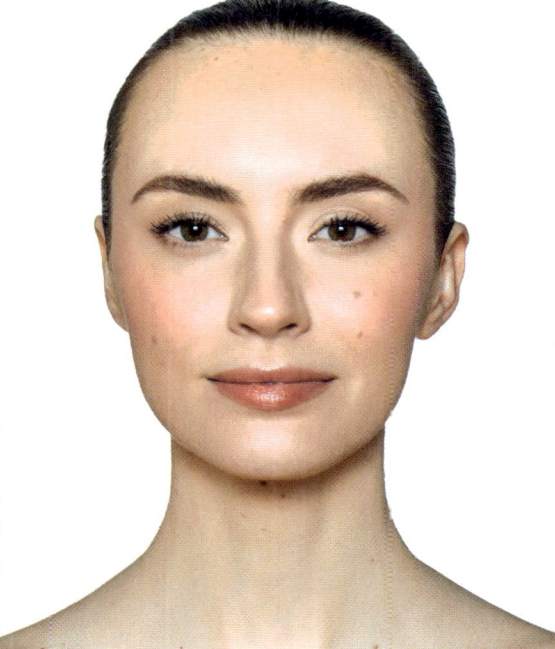

1 Open your eyes
Keeping the rest of your face relaxed, open your eyes as much as possible and hold them wide open for a second. Then relax for a second.

2 Repeat
Repeat this movement for 1 minute, avoiding engaging your forehead at all times.

TIP

Place your fingertips on your forehead while doing the exercise. If you feel any movement or tension under your fingers, slow down the motion and reduce the intensity until your forehead stays completely relaxed.

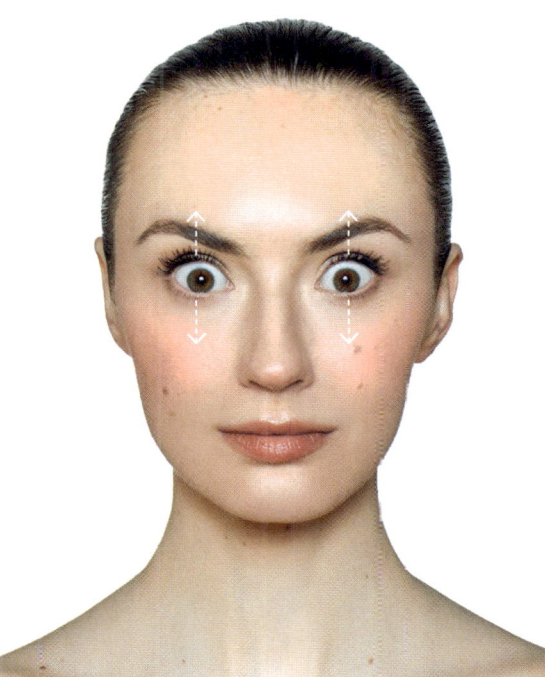

THE METHOD & MOVEMENTS

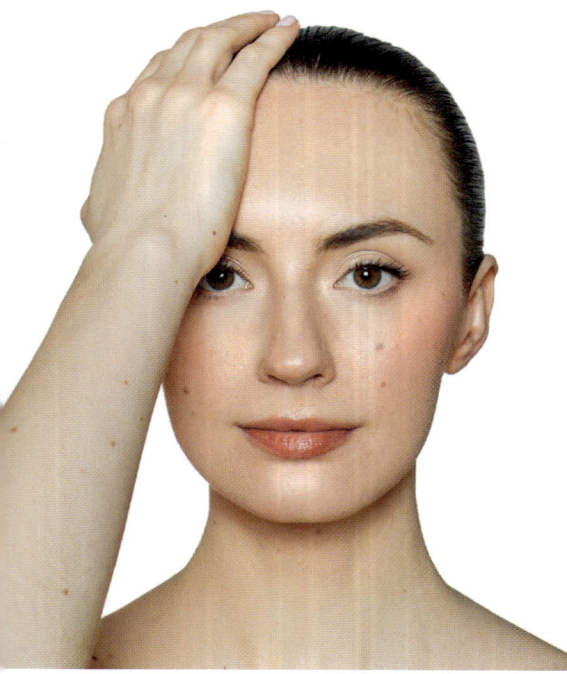

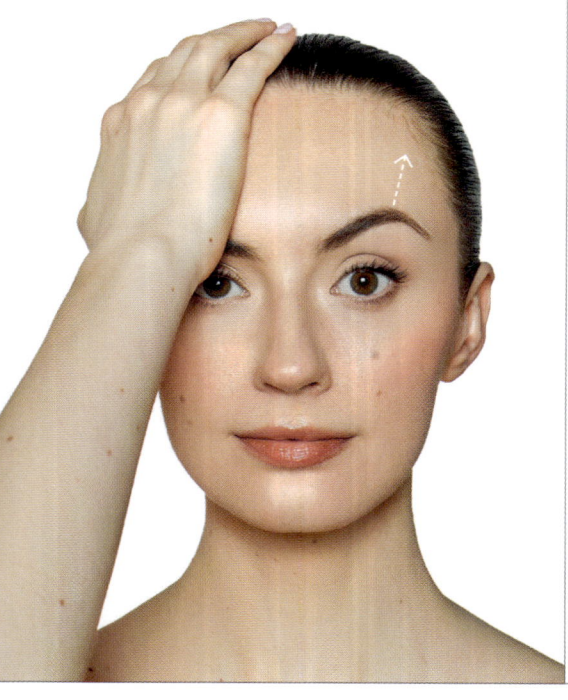

 1 MIN

The Eye Symmetry Workout

Awaken your eyes & improve their symmetry

This move helps to retrain and reawaken the muscles around your less active eye, creating better balance between both sides of your face, which leads to powerful shifts in symmetry.

1 Find your weaker side
To begin, determine which is your strongest, or slightly less lifted eye. You can do this by looking in the mirror, or, if you can't see a difference, raise the eyebrows one at a time to see which one feels the weakest and least flexible.

2 Place your palm
Place your palm on the stronger eyebrow and the forehead above it. Press slightly to hold it firm throughout this exercise, so that it doesn't move.

3 Raise the other eyebrow
Slowly raise and drop the weaker eyebrow, reducing the range of motion if your forehead begins to wrinkle.

4 Repeat
Repeat for 1 minute.

👀 1 MIN

The Pencil Push Up

Strengthen your eye endurance & focus

This eye coordination drill strengthens the muscles responsible for focus. It's a effective way to boost eye endurance and clarity, which is especially helpful if you spend long hours on screens.

1 Grab a pencil
Grab a pencil, pen, makeup brush, or chopstick.

2 Hold
Hold the object in front of your face.

3 Slowly move it
Slowly move the object towards, and then away from your face, focusing your eyes on the pointy tip of the object as it moves to constantly readjust your focus, and strengthen your eyes.

4 Continue
Continue focusing on the moving object for 1 minute.

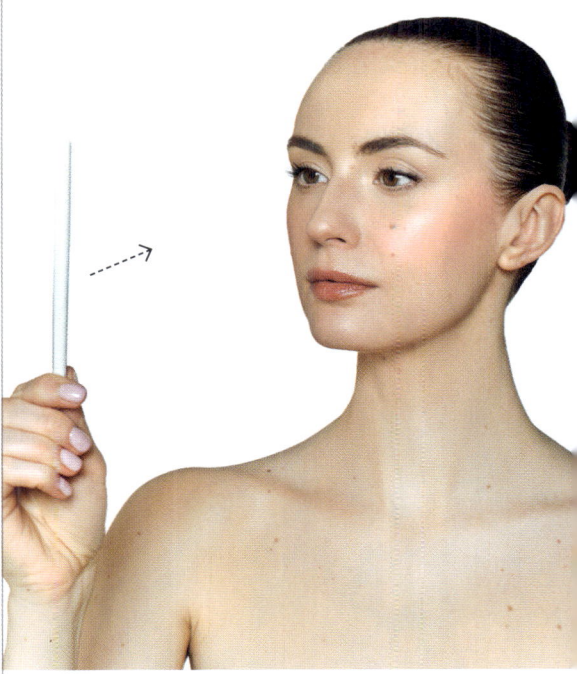

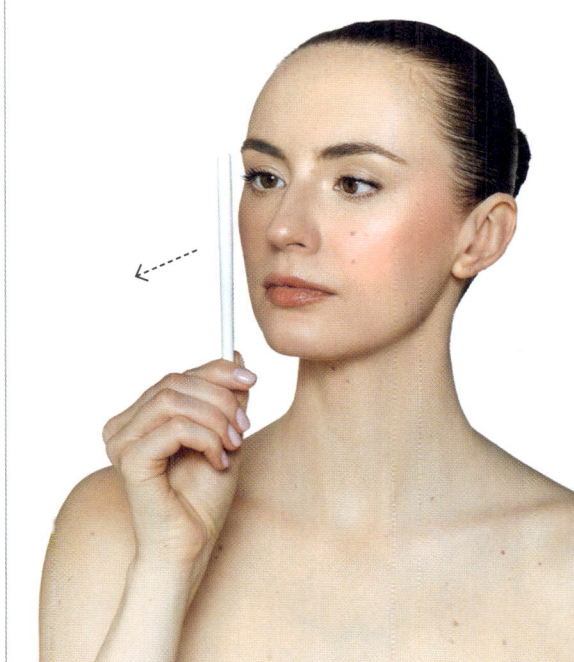

THE METHOD & MOVEMENTS

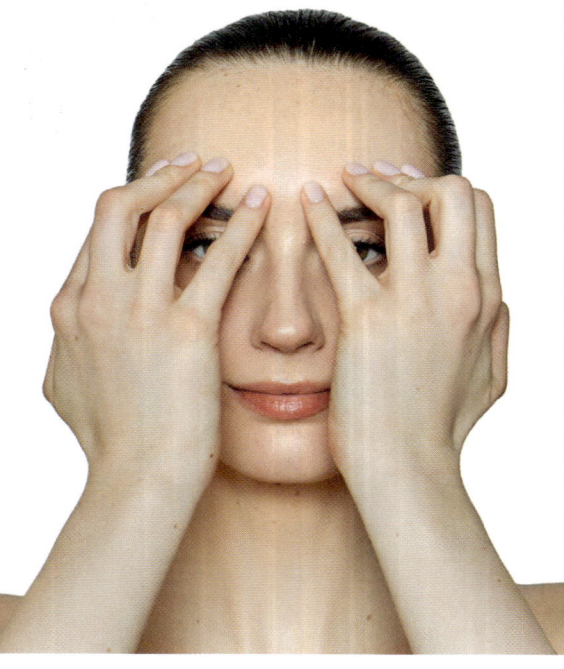
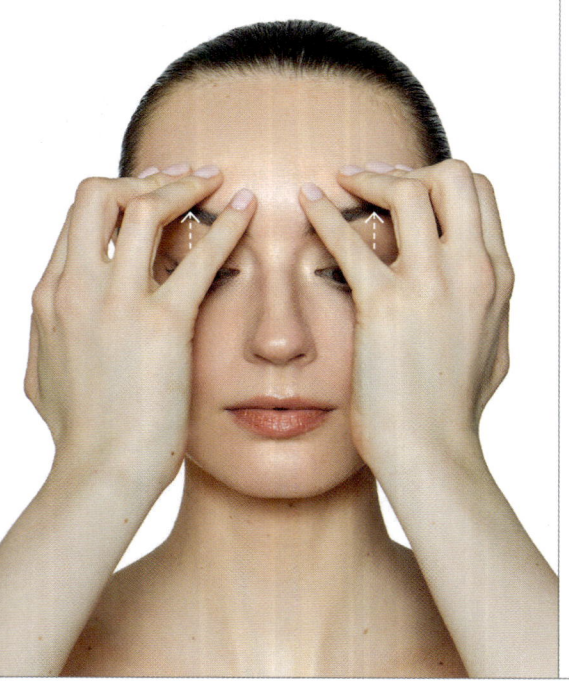

 1 M N

Forehead Resistance Training

Soothe & strengthen your forehead

This exercise retrains your facial coordination, teaching you how to lift the brows using only the right muscles while keeping the forehead smooth and relaxed.

1   **Place your fingertips**
Place your fingertips on your forehead, just above each eyebrow, pressing into each fingertip to form resistance.

2   **Raise your brows**
Raise your eyebrows, hold them up for a second, then release them, ensuring you're not wrinkling your forehead. If your forehead wrinkles, reduce the resistance in the hands, raise the eyebrows less high, or move slower.

3   **Repeat**
Repeat for 1 minute.

1 MIN

The Forehead Finger Push Up

Smooth your forehead & reduce lines

This gentle strength-training move helps retrain your upper facial muscles to lift without overusing your forehead. It's ideal for reducing lines caused by habitual brow movement.

1 Place and press your fingers
Place your index fingers horizontally onto your forehead, just above your eyebrows. Slightly press the eyebrows down.

2 Raise your brows
Raise your eyebrows, hold them up for a second, then release them. The movement in your eyebrows should raise your fingers up and down. Avoid frowning and keeping gentle pressure in the fingers to form resistance.

3 Repeat
Repeat for 1 minute.

> **TIP**
> Focus on slow, isolated lifts. Imagine you're waking up sleepy muscles beneath the brow. Less is more here.

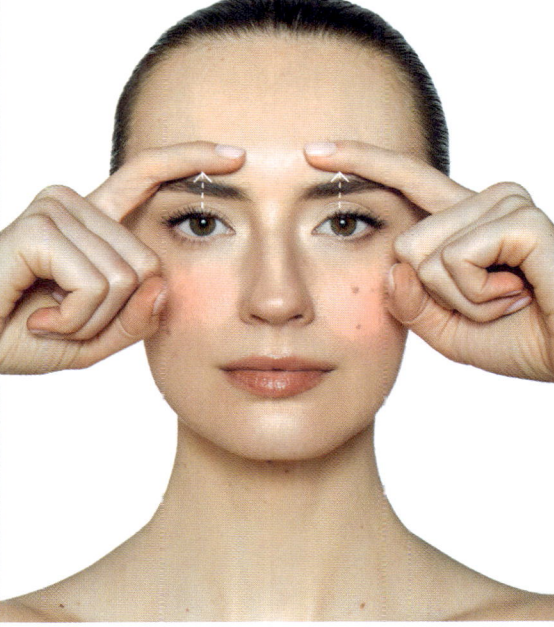

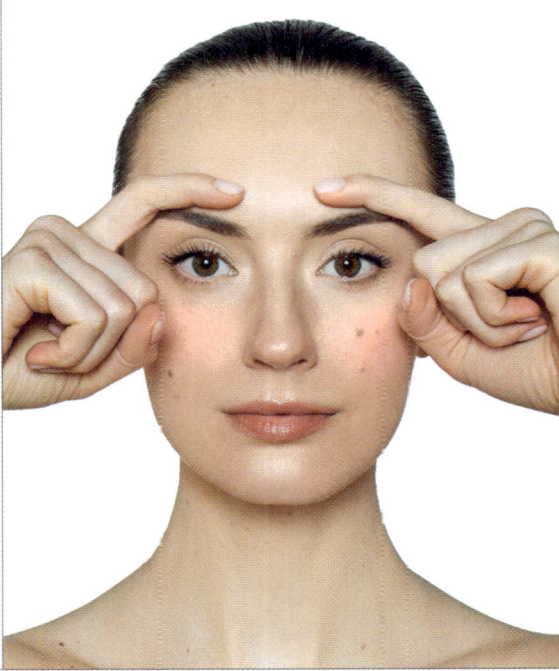

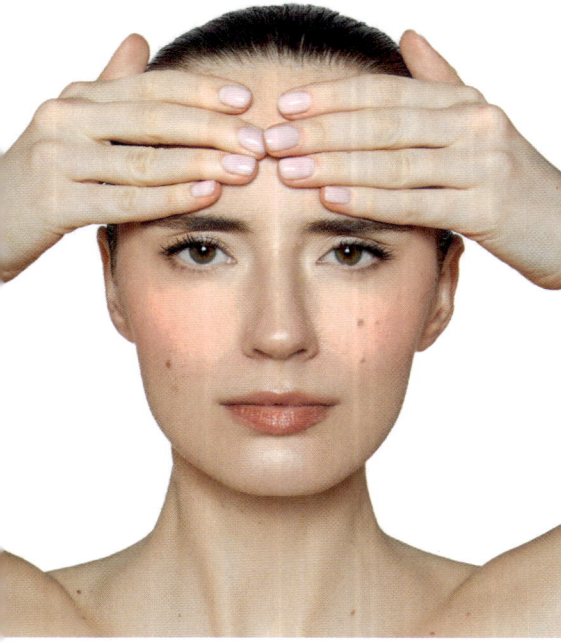

 1 MIN

The Forehead Smoother

Calm your mind & soften forehead lines

This exercise helps release forehead tension, reducing horizontal lines and promoting smoother, more expressive movement. It's ideal after a long day of thinking, frowning, or screen time.

1 Place your hands
Place your fingers horizontally across your forehead, and gently press them down towards your eyebrows.

2 Raise your brows
Slowly raise and release your eyebrows while keeping the pressure in your fingers, which should act as resistance against your eyebrows, and prevent wrinkles on your forehead from forming.

3 Repeat
Repeat this raising and releasing motion for 1 minute.

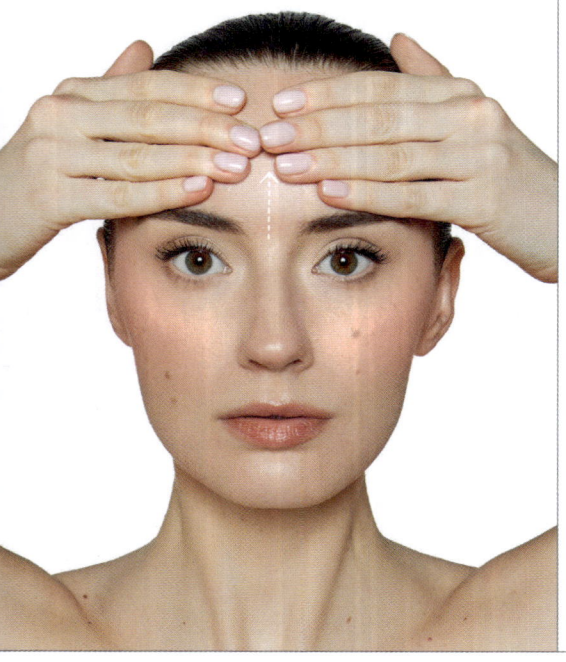

> **TIP**
> Slow down the movement if you see wrinkles starting to form. Hold them firm with your hands.

FACE YOGA

1 MIN

The Happy Booster

Activate your muscles & boost your mood

This technique supports facial symmetry, lifts the muscles that contribute to a youthful expression, and encourages the release of "happy chemicals" such as dopamine and serotonin.

1 **Smile**
Think of something pleasant that makes you happy, and create your biggest smile. You can smile with your mouth open or closed, or alternate between the two. Look into the mirror while doing this and observe your smile symmetry. Avoid frowning and smile with both sides of your mouth equally to improve your facial symmetry. Keep smiling for the entire minute even if it feels silly. You will feel the effect later in the day.

TIP
To increase your happiness while doing this exercise even more, think of something you are grateful for, look at yourself, or give yourself a compliment.

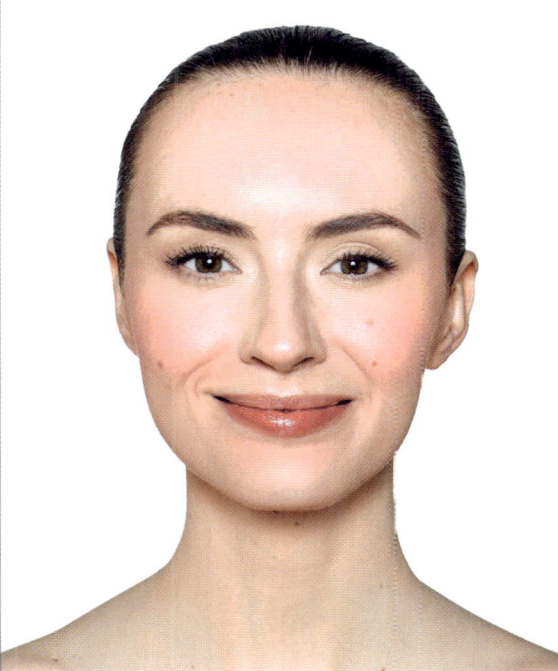

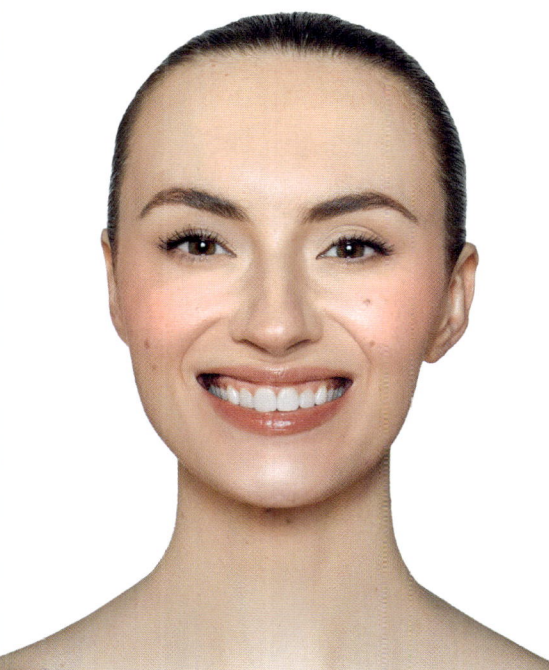

THE METHOD & MOVEMENTS

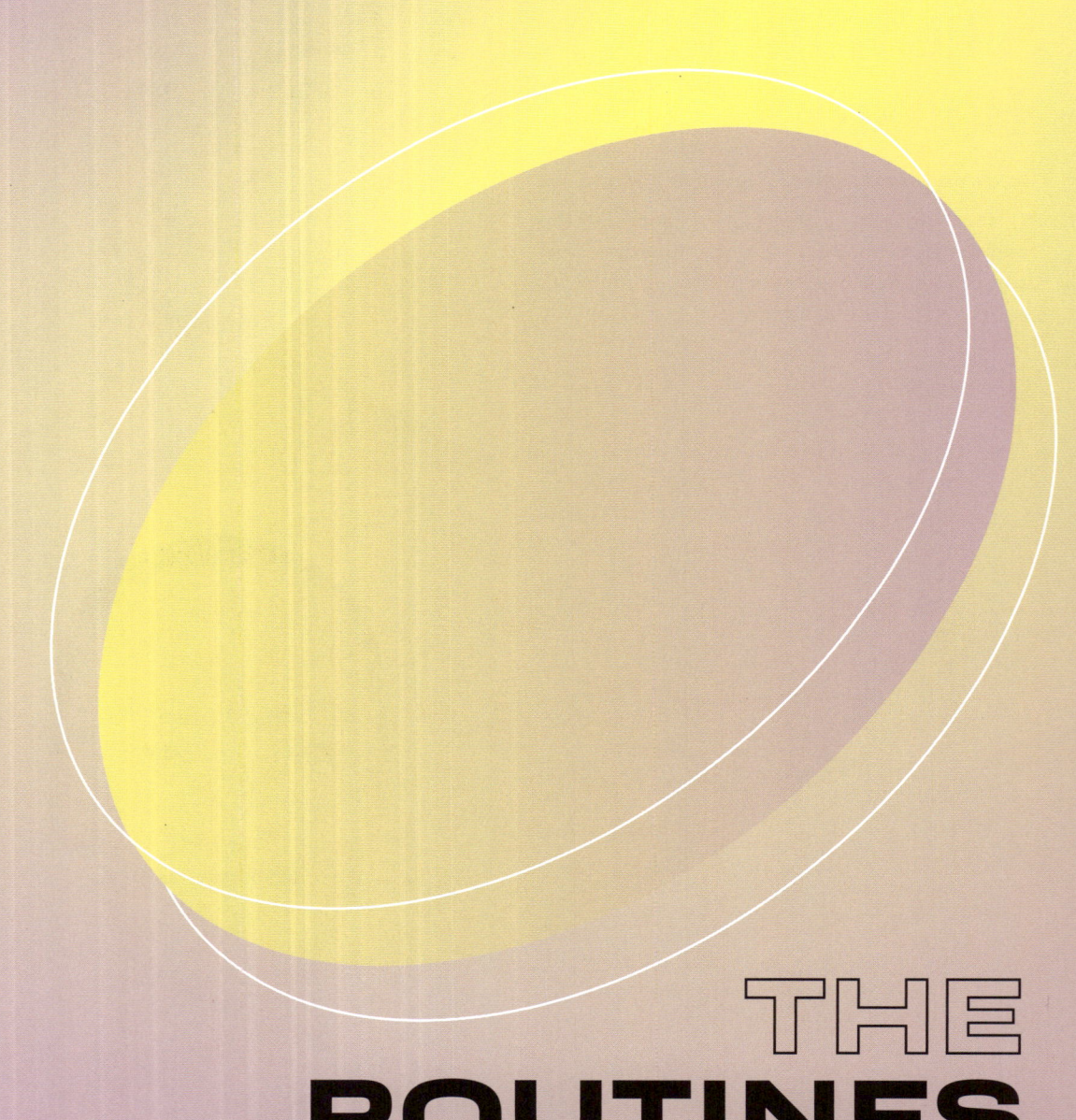

These routines offer a simple, effective way to take action based on what you see and feel, whether you're looking to lift tired eyes, balance asymmetry, or define your jawline.

Not every routine in this chapter follows the full Phase 1-2-3 system in strict order, and that's intentional. These are focused, accessible sequences designed to target common concerns, whether you're short on time or looking for a specific result.

For optimal, long-term transformation, I always recommend incorporating the full method regularly, as that's the foundation for real, lasting change. The shorter routines, like those in this chapter, are incredibly useful as daily add-ons or mood-based boosters.

Combat Tired Eyes

Refresh, lift, & awaken your eyes naturally

11 MIN

1

The Big 6 Lymphatic Activation
p.52

What it does Clears drainage pathways so puffiness can flow out effectively.

How Massage key points in sequence: collarbones, neck, underarms, belly, groin, behind knees.

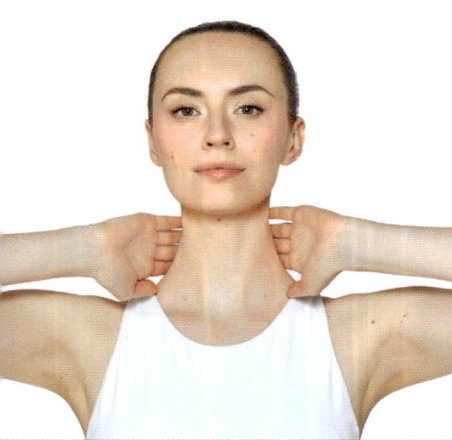

2

The Eye Depuffer
p.97

What it does Clears drainage pathways so puffiness can flow out effectively.

How Press key points gently along the eye socket (inner brow, outer brow, temples).

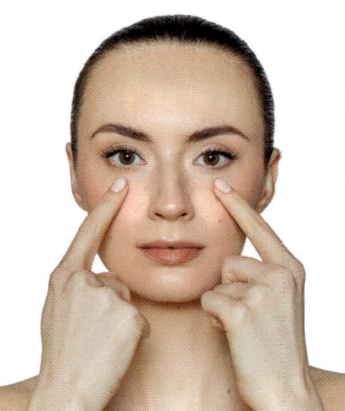

3

The Upper Eyelid Depuffer
p.95

What it does Stimulates drainage and reduces puffiness.

How Gently massage under the brow bone, moving outwards.

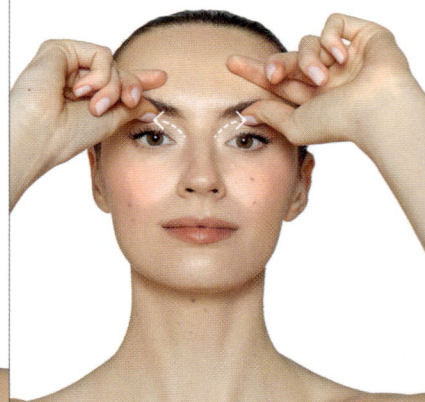

WHEN TO PRACTISE THIS ROUTINE

When fatigue, long days, or poor circulation dull your gaze, this reset clears puffiness and strengthens eye muscles to revive tired eyes, leaving them brighter, open, and naturally refreshed.

4

The Cat Eye Lift
p.151

What it does Instantly lifts outer eye corners and reduces sagging.

How Press palms into your temples, lift the face slightly, and squint down.

5

Eye Gymnastics
p.147

What it does Boosts blood flow and reduces eye fatigue.

How Look up and down, then side to side, slowly and with control.

6

The Under-Eye Push Up
p.148

What it does Activates the lower-eye muscles to firm and lift.

How Press gently with your middle and index fingers at the corners of the eyes, then squint up.

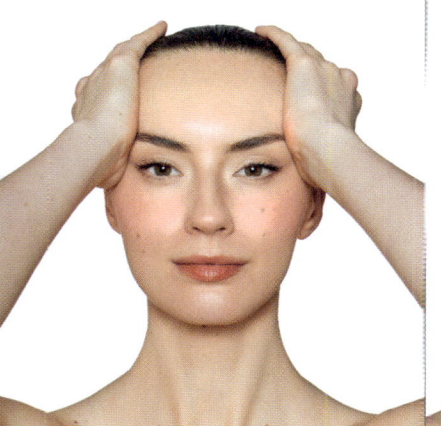
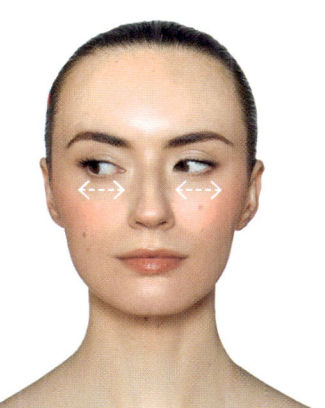
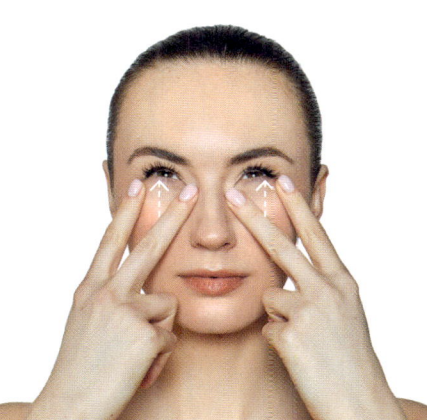

THE ROUTINES

Combat Puffy Eyes

Depuff, refresh, & brighten your eye area

10 MIN

1

The Big 6 Lymphatic Activation
p.52

What it does Clears drainage pathways so puffiness can flow out effectively.

How Massage key points in sequence: collarbones, neck, underarms, belly, groin, behind knees.

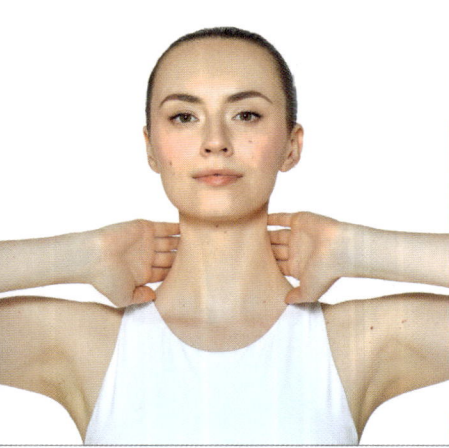

2

The Eye Knuckle Glider
p.96

What it does Releases tension and encourages drainage around the eyes.

How Glide soft knuckles slowly along the orbital bone from the inner to outer corner, keeping steady contact.

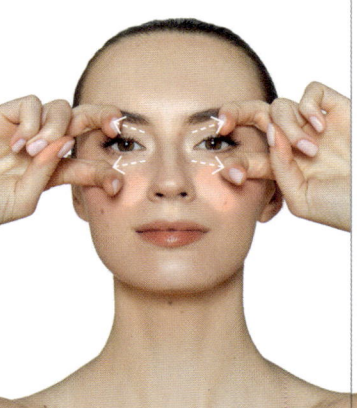

3

The Eye Depuffer
p.97

What it does Combats general eye puffiness.

How Press key points gently along the eye socket (inner brow, outer brow, temples).

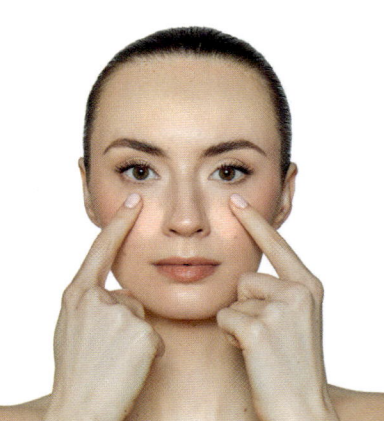

> **WHEN TO PRACTISE THIS ROUTINE**
>
> *When mornings, travel, or long days leave your eyes swollen and heavy, these techniques clear lymph pathways and reawaken the eye area. Just 10 minutes can refresh your gaze and bring back brightness naturally.*

4

The Upper Eyelid Depuffer
p.95

What it does Stimulates drainage and reduces puffiness.

How Gently massage under the brow bone, moving outwards.

5

The Under-Eye Zigzag
p.99

What it does Releases micro-tension and softens the under-eye area for smoother, depuffed skin.

How Create small zigzag motions along the under-eye, moving outwards towards the temple.

6

The Eye Roll Lift
p.101

What it does Lifts and resets fascia at the outer eye and temple to reduce tension and sagging.

How Gently pinch outer-eye tissue, and roll diagonally up towards the temple and outer hairline.

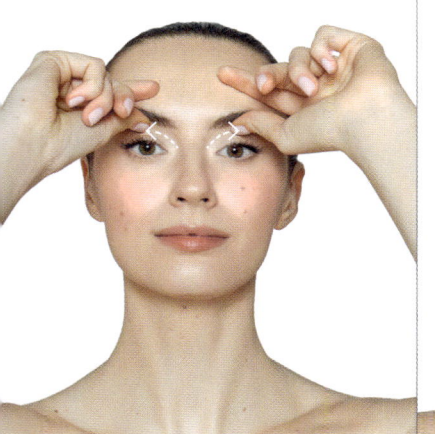
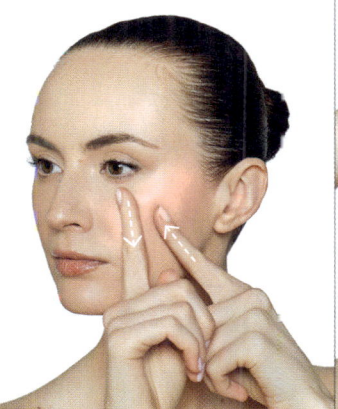
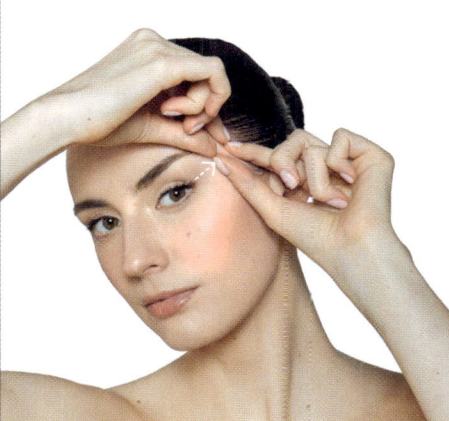

THE ROUTINES

Combat Drooping Eyelids

Lift, tone, & brighten your upper-eye area

5.5 MIN

1

The Forehead Smoother
p.160

What it does Trains your brows and eyes to lift without engaging the forehead.

How Place hands on your forehead as light resistance. Slowly raise your eyebrows. Hold and release.

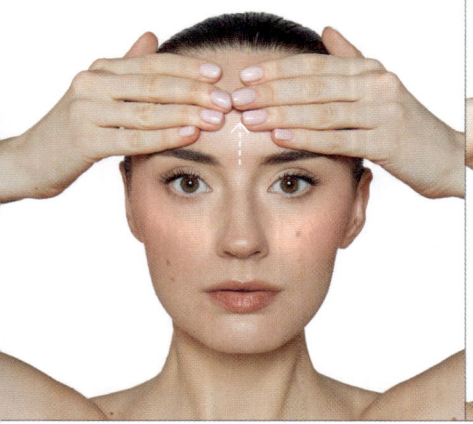

2

The Brow Lift Glide
p.93

What it does Lifts and reawakens the upper eye area by releasing fascia tension beneath the brow.

How Anchor one brow with your fingertips. Glide the knuckles or fingertips of the other hand slowly upwards from the brow to the hairline.

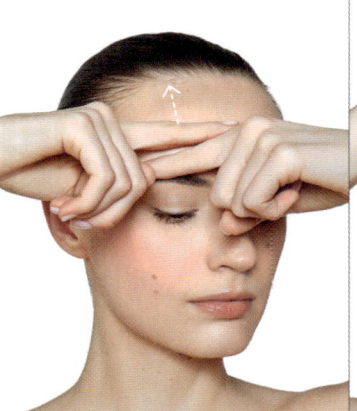

3

The Eye Roll Lift
p.101

What it does Releases fascia tension and resets the outer-eye and temple area.

How Gently pinch outer-eye tissue, and roll diagonally up towards the temple and outer hairline.

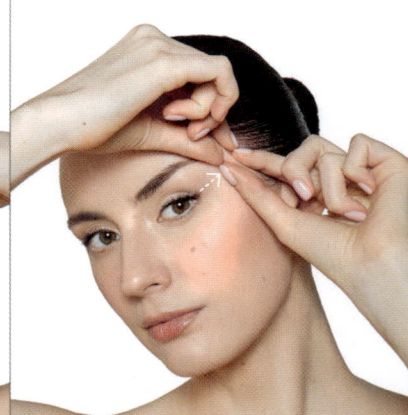

WHEN TO PRACTISE THIS ROUTINE

When eyes feel tired, heavy, or lose their natural openness, this sequence awakens upper eyelid muscles and fascia. A gentle lift restores brightness and rebalances posture so your gaze looks alert, refreshed, and naturally lifted.

4

The Under-Eye Toner
p.149

What it does Strengthens and lifts the lower-eye area.

How Place hands on temples for a gentle lift. Look up and squint with just the under-eyes, avoiding forehead engagement.

5

The Secret Spy
p.154

What it does Activates the ring muscle of the eye for tone and lift.

How Form circles around your eyes with thumbs and index fingers (like spyglasses). Alternate between squinting and widening the eyes slowly.

6

The Eyelid Stretch
p.153

What it does Stretches and depuffs the upper eyelids.

How Place palms above brows, lift gently, look down, and blink slowly to feel the stretch.

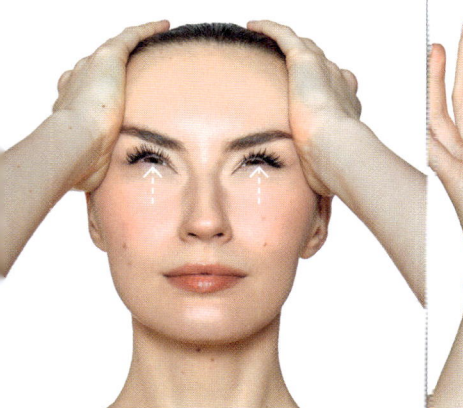
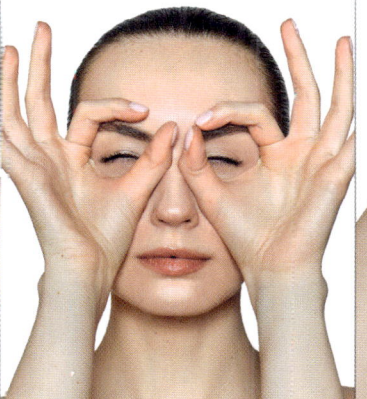
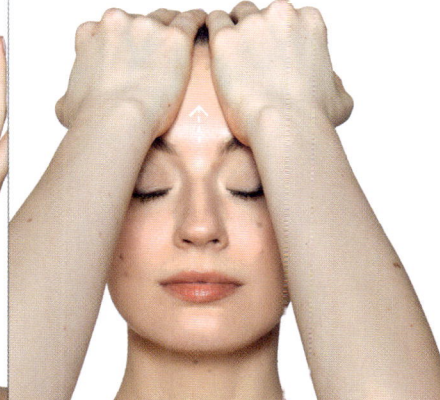

Combat Frown Lines

Soften tension, smooth lines, & restore a calm expression

7 MIN

1

The Scalp Shake
p.80

What it does Re eases tension at the scalp to ease tightness across the forehead and brow.

How Gently grasp sections of your scalp and shake from side to side, loosening the tissue beneath.

2

The Forehead Massage
p.88

What it does Relaxes overactive forehead muscles and smooths lines.

How Use fingers to glide in small zigzags or long, slow strokes across the forehead.

3

The Forehead Knuckle Glider
p.89

What it does Lifts and resets tight fascia across the forehead.

How Glide soft knuckles slowly upwards from brows to hairline.

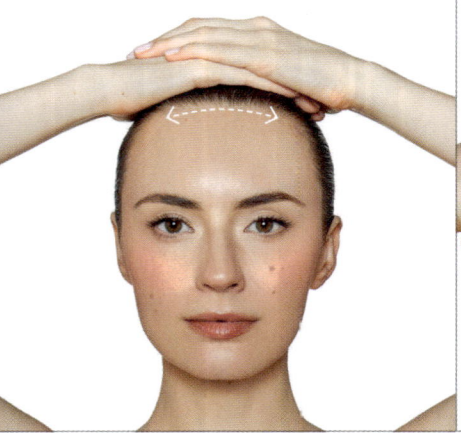
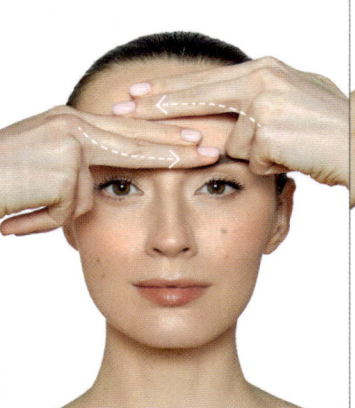
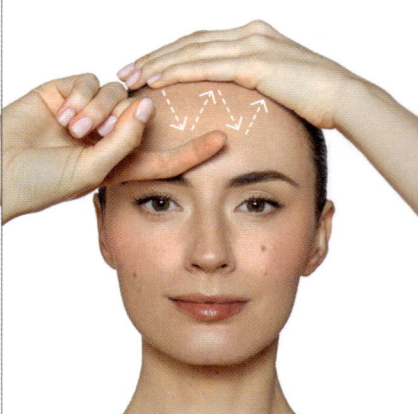

WHEN TO PRACTISE THIS ROUTINE

When stress or focus etches lines between your brows, these moves calm the forehead fascia and retrain expression patterns. With regular practice, tension softens, your brow opens, and your face reflects ease again.

4

The Frowning X
p.91

What it does Builds awareness and control to prevent habitual frowning.

How Cross your index and middle fingers over the space between your brows in an "X" shape. Try to frown gently while your fingers hold the muscles firmly in place, preventing movement. Hold and release repeatedly.

5

The 11 Line Eraser
p.92

What it does Releases tension and smooths vertical lines between the brows.

How Gently pinch each eyebrow and massage in slow circular motions along the brow. Then pinch the space between the brows and massage outwards towards the temples.

6

The Forehead Tap
p.87

What it does Boosts circulation and relaxes overactive forehead muscles.

How Lightly tap across the forehead, moving from the centre out to the temples.

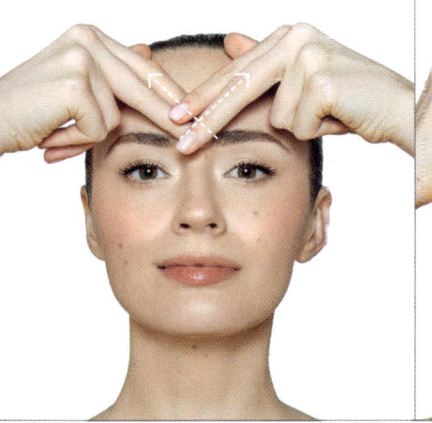
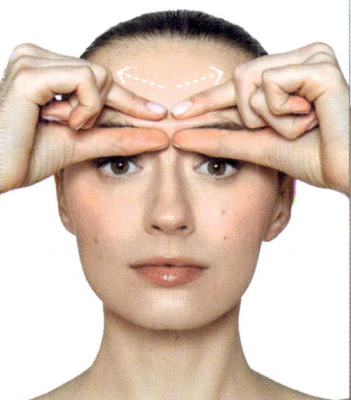
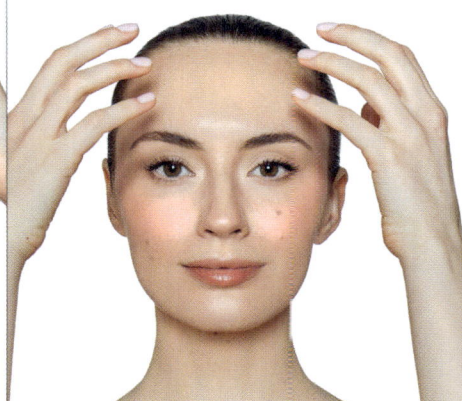

THE ROUTINES

Combat Sagging Cheeks

Lift, tone, & sculpt your cheeks

6.5 MIN

1

The Cheekbone Sculpt
p.104

What it does Releases tension, boosts circulation, and defines the cheekbones.

How Use index fingers or knuckles to press next to the nostrils, then under the cheeks, and towards the ends of the cheekbones near the ears.

2

The Cheeky Booster
p.146

What it does Lifts the cheeks and enhances facial symmetry.

How Smile with your mouth closed, keeping both sides even. Place fingertips on the apples of your cheeks and hold the smile.

3

The Cheek Push & Pull
p.142

What it does Strengthens the cheeks and mouth area while smoothing nasolabial folds.

How Place one hand on your cheek, gently lifting. Pucker lips and blow air towards the opposite side. Repeat on both sides.

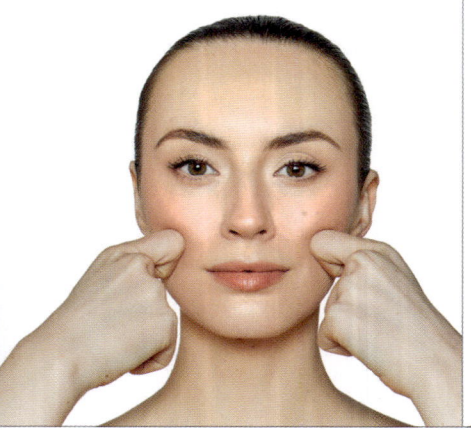
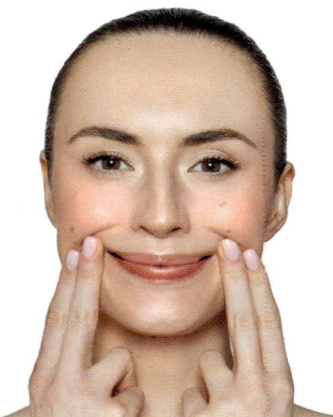
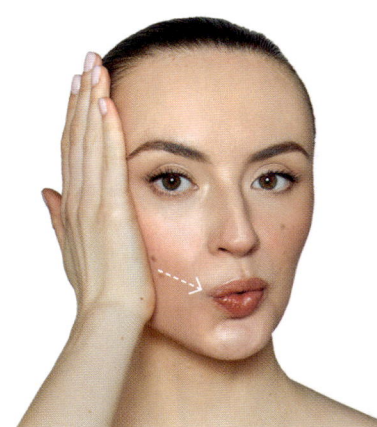

WHEN TO PRACTISE THIS ROUTINE

When cheeks feel heavy, lips droop, or symmetry fades, this sequence redefines your mid-face. By activating cheek muscles and fascia, it restores lift and lightness, helping your expression stay energized and youthful.

4

The Cheeky Lift
p.137

What it does Builds cheek muscle strength and softens nasolabial folds.

How Cover teeth with lips and smile tightly. Place hands at sides of face and lift slightly, keeping tension in the cheek.

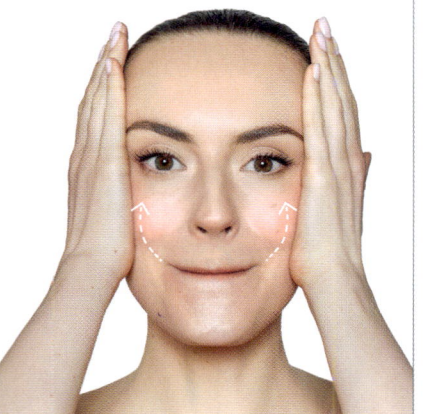

5

The Smiling "O"
p.144

What it does Tones cheeks and lips while supporting symmetry.

How Form an "O" with your lips and smile simultaneously, lifting from the cheeks.

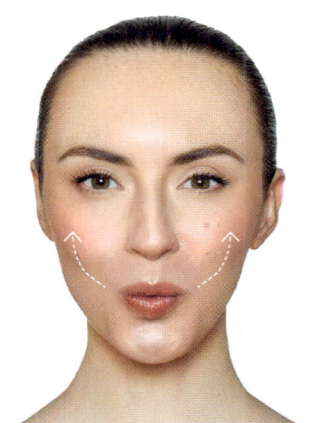

6

The Blow Up
p.135

What it does Strengthens and plumps cheeks, smoothing folds.

How Fill mouth with air and move it in a circular path: left cheek, upper lip, right cheek, lower lip.

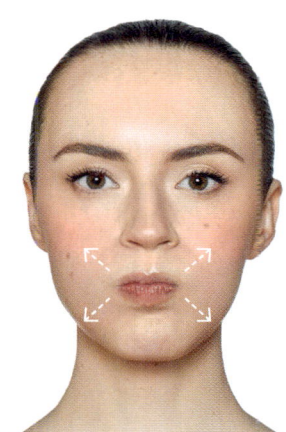

Combat Smile Lines

Soften nasolabial folds, release tension, & support a lifted, youthful expression

6 MIN

1

The Masseter Relaxer
p.83

What it does Releases jaw tension that can pull down the mouth corners and deepen folds.

How Glide knuckles slowly from in front of the ear down towards the jawline, with mouth slightly open.

2

The Nasolabial Fold Eraser
p.103

What it does Releases tension along the folds and softens the muscle patterns that deepen lines.

How Massage next to nostrils in small circles for 30 seconds. Then glide fingers up and down the sides of the nose in circular motions for 30 seconds.

3

The Pouty Lip
p.110

What it does Plumps the lips, smooths edges, and releases tension that pulls down the mouth corners.

How Hold lips between index fingers and thumbs. Move your fingers side to side along lips, pressing firmly and focusing on corners.

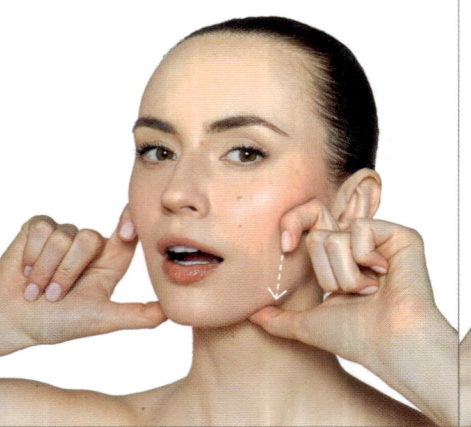
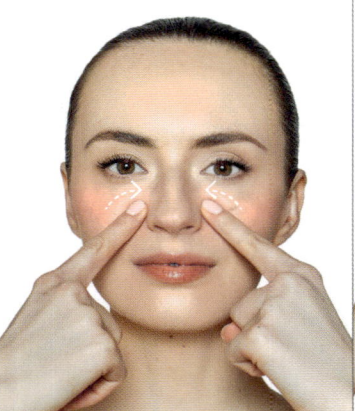
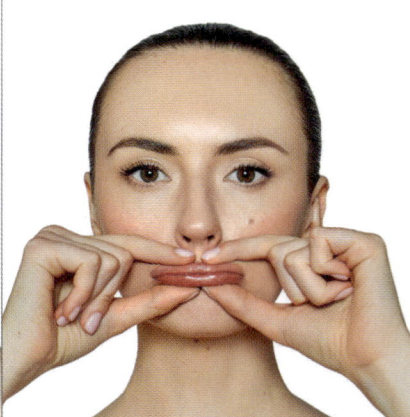

FACE YOGA

WHEN TO PRACTISE THIS ROUTINE

When tension deepens folds or lips lose vitality, these techniques blend strength and release. The focus is not erasing lines, but softening habits and re-energizing tissues so your expression feels supported, lifted, and truly alive.

4

The Mouth Relaxer
p.109

What it does Lets go of built-up mouth and jaw tension.

How Blow out through the mouth with heavy breath, letting lips vibrate in a "Brrrrrrrrr" sound.

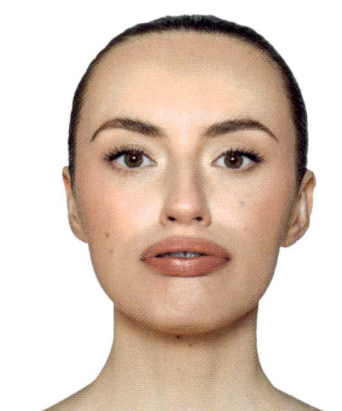

5

The Blow Up
p.135

What it does Strengthens cheeks and smooths nasolabial folds.

How Fill your mouth with air and move it in a circular pattern: left cheek, upper lip, right cheek, lower lip. Reverse halfway through.

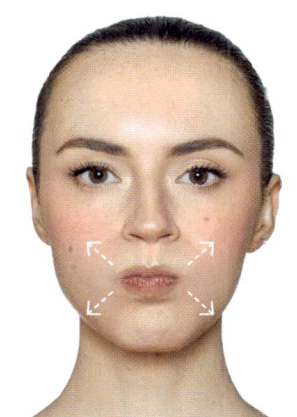

6

The Roundabout
p.136

What it does Tones and strengthens the mouth area to soften smile lines.

How Press your tongue into one corner inside your mouth and circle it around the mouth, pressing into the skin. Reverse direction after 45 seconds.

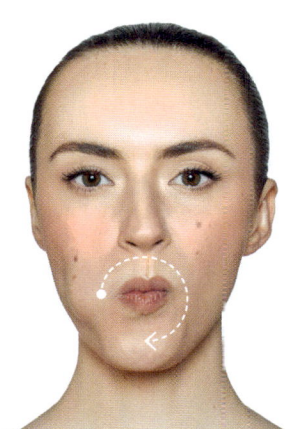

Combat Thinning Lips

Plump, rebalance, & soften the mouth area

6 MIN

1

The Laugh Line & Cheek Lift
p.141

What it does Supports fuller lips by lifting the cheeks that frame them and easing nasolabial folds.

How Cover teeth with lips and smile tightly. Place fingertips at nasolabial folds and lift slightly as you hold the cheek lift.

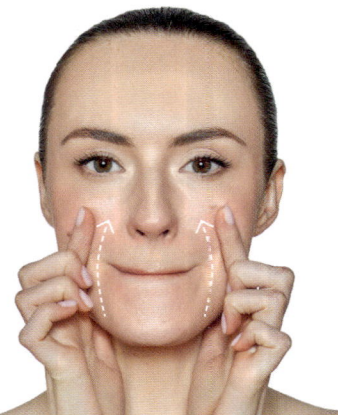

2

The Droopy Mouth Release
p.112

What it does Frees the downwards pull at the mouth corners that thins and turns lips under.

How Place an index finger at one mouth corner; glide slowly downwards along the depressor muscle towards the jaw.

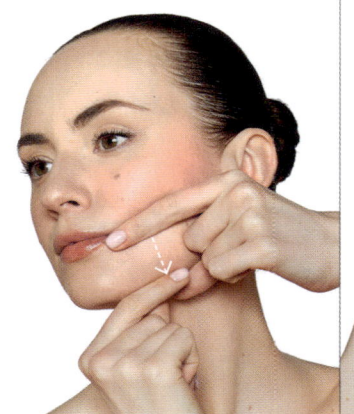

3

The Kiss Shaper
p.129

What it does Builds balanced lip projection and strengthens circular lip muscles.

How Frame your mouth with index fingers and thumbs. Form a controlled "kiss" and press gently into your fingers for resistance.

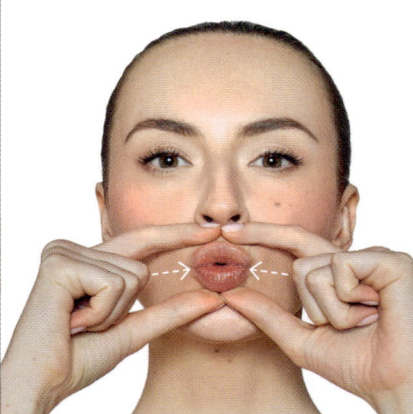

FACE YOGA

WHEN TO PRACTISE THIS ROUTINE

When lips feel flat, compressed, or lose softness, these moves reawaken circulation and muscle tone. Rather than fillers, you use your own hands to restore volume, redefine shape, and keep lips supple and expressive.

4

The Lip Liner
p.111

What it does Stimulates circulation at the lip edge for natural definition and colour.

How Using thumb and index finger, lightly pinch around the entire edge of the lips.

5

The Pouty Lip
p.110

What it does Deeply releases tension and plumps lip tissue (especially at the corners, where thinning starts).

How Hold lips between index fingers and thumbs. Move fingers from side to side along lips, pressing firmly and focusing on corners.

6

The Mouth Relaxer
p.109

What it does Lets go of hidden tension that compresses the lips and lowers their volume.

How Blow out through the mouth with heavy breath, letting lips vibrate in a "Brrrrrrrrr" sound.

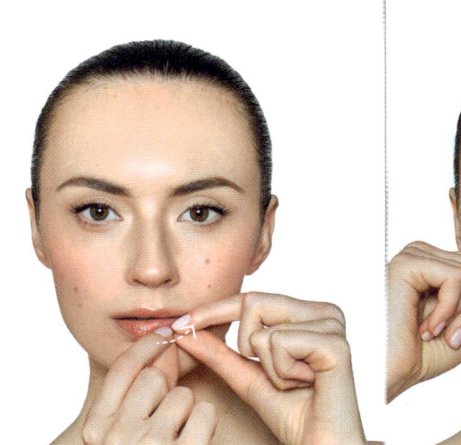
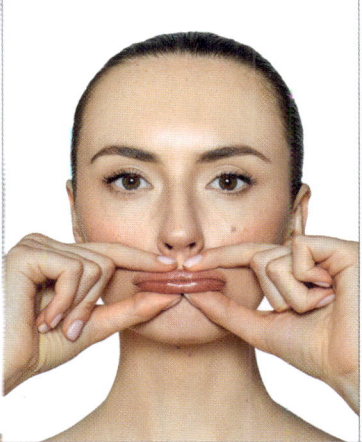
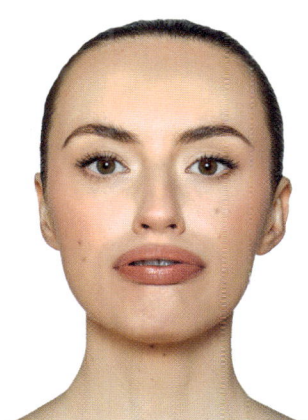

THE ROUTINES

Combat a Drooping Mouth

Lift mouth corners, soften tension, & rebalance your expression

6 MIN

1

The Droopy Mouth Release
p.112

What it does Releases muscle tension that pulls the mouth corners downwards.

How Place fingertips just outside the corners of your lips. Massage upwards in small circles, then glide slightly out towards the temples.

2

The Happy Booster
p.161

What it does Builds strength in the muscles that lift the mouth corners.

How Smile gently with lips closed and place fingers at the corners of your mouth. Apply light upwards resistance while maintaining the smile.

3

The Smiling Push Up
p.131

What it does Trains the corners of the mouth to lift evenly and naturally.

How Smile as wide as you can with lips closed. Press the corners of your mouth upwards with your fingers or visualize the upward motion. Hold the tension and repeat.

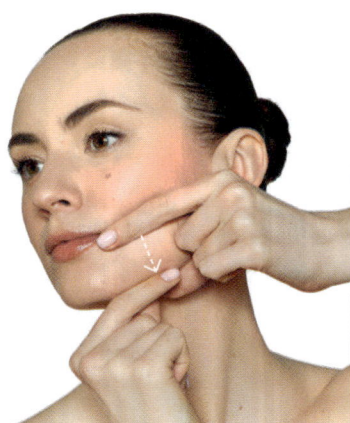
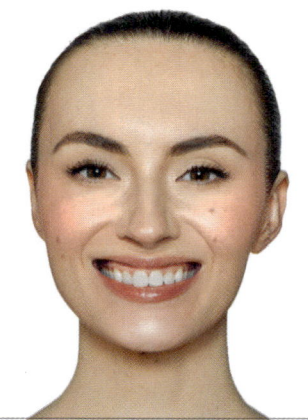
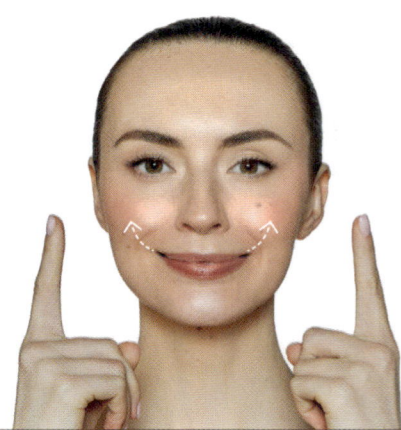

WHEN TO PRACTISE THIS ROUTINE

When corners pull down from tension, sadness, or habit, this series brings gentle strength back to the lips and surrounding muscles. Small, consistent practice can rebalance your smile and lift your mood from within.

4

The Symmetrical Smile Line
p.134

What it does Supports balanced smiling.

How Place a clean pen or makeup brush between your teeth, cover it with your lips, and smile with both corners evenly lifted.

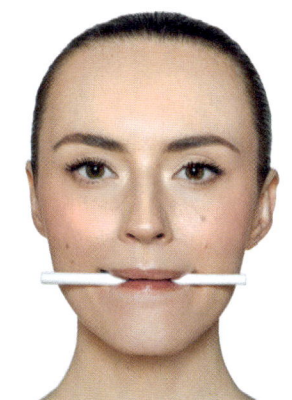

5

The Tongue Dancer
p.133

What it does Tones cheek and mouth muscles and lifts the corners from within.

How Smile widely with both corners lifted. Stick your tongue out and slide it to one side of your mouth, tipping slightly up. Hold, then move to the other side.

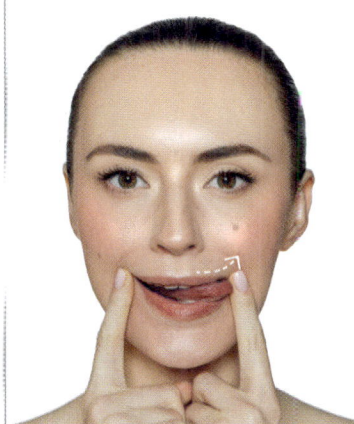

6

The Mouth Relaxer
p.109

What it does Releases lingering tension in the lips and jaw that pulls the face downwards.

How Blow out through the mouth with heavy breath, letting lips vibrate in a "Brrrrrrrrr" sound.

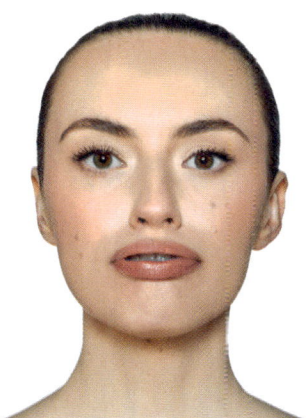

Combat Jaw Tension

10 MIN

Release clenching, soften your jawline, & restore flow

1

The Wow
p.82

What it does Warms up facial muscles, releases jaw tension, and boosts mood.

How Slowly and exaggeratedly say "Wow," starting with a small "O" shape and expanding as wide as possible without frowning.

2

The Masseter Relaxer
p.83

What it does Softens the masseter muscle and helps release deep jaw tension.

How Glide knuckles slowly from in front of the ear down towards the jawline, with the mouth slightly open.

3

The Diagonal Masseter Opener
p.84

What it does Releases tension and encourages lift and softness.

How Glide fingers or knuckles diagonally from under the cheekbone down to the jaw angle.

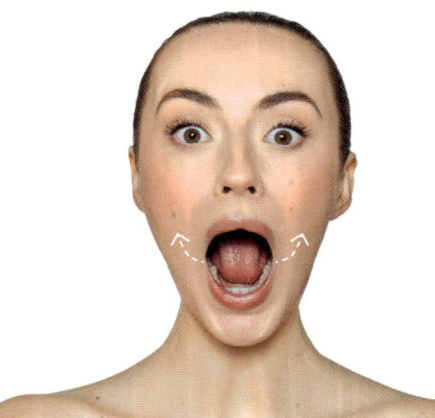
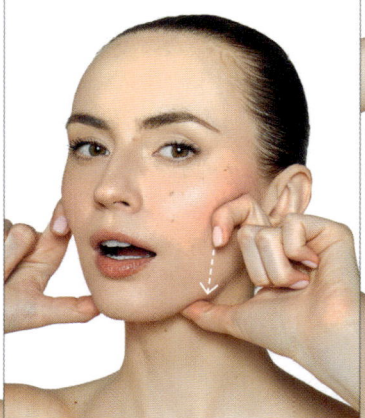
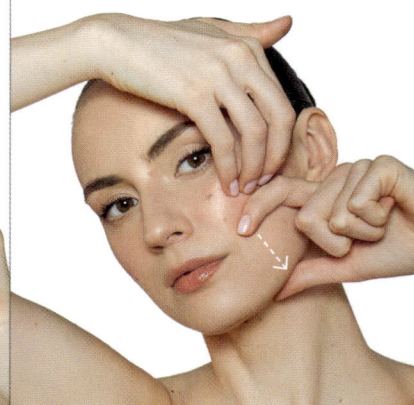

WHEN TO PRACTISE THIS ROUTINE

When clenching, grinding, or stress hardens the jaw, this reset unblocks the masseter and surrounding fascia. These moves soften tension patterns, refine jaw contours, and restore ease, freeing your face to move fluidly again.

4

The Buccal Massage Release
p.85

What it does Unlocks tension for deep muscle and fascia release.

How With clean hands, place thumb inside cheek, and using outside fingers, knead along the masseter.

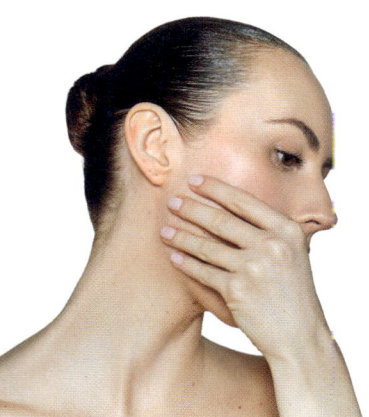

5

The Masseter Rolls
p.86

What it does Lifts and rehydrates tight jaw fascia for improved mobility and softness.

How Gently grab jawline tissue and roll it slowly upwards towards the temples.

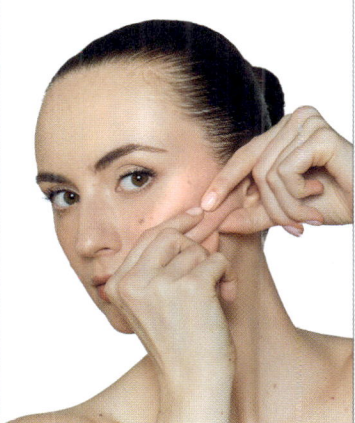

6

The Jawline Hook
p.115

What it does Releases tension along the jawline and supports lymphatic drainage.

How Hook index fingers onto jawline at the chin and press thumbs under the jawbone. Hold for 20 seconds, moving from chin to mid-jaw, then to near the ears.

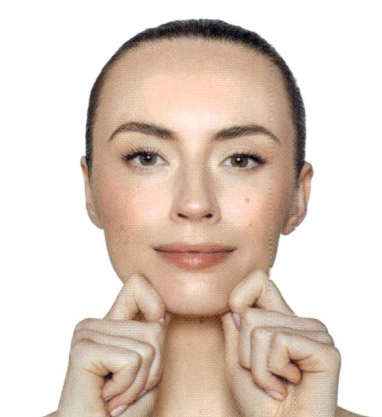

THE ROUTINES

Combat a Double Chin

6 MIN

Strengthen, sculpt, & elongate the neck, chin, & jawline

1

The Neck Tap
p.55

What it does Stimulates lymph flow, stretches the neck, and supports jawline definition.

How Tilt your head, look up, and gently tap from the top of your neck towards your shoulder with the opposite hand. Switch sides after 30 seconds.

2

The SCM Release
p.76

What it does Frees tension in the neck muscle that can contribute to a double chin.

How Grasp the SCM between your fingers, tilt your head for a deeper stretch, and massage slowly along its length.

3

The Jawline Hook
p.115

What it does Releases jaw tension and supports lymphatic drainage along the jawline.

How Hook your thumbs under the jaw and index fingers onto your jawline at the chin. Hold, then move along the jawline towards the ears in sections.

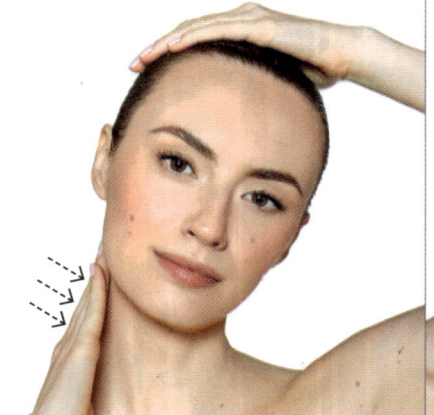
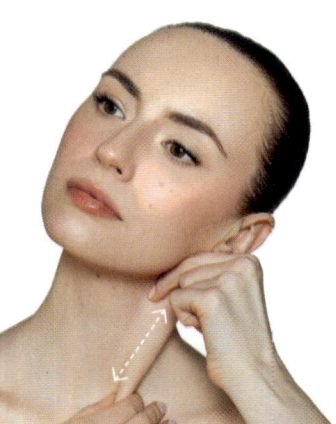
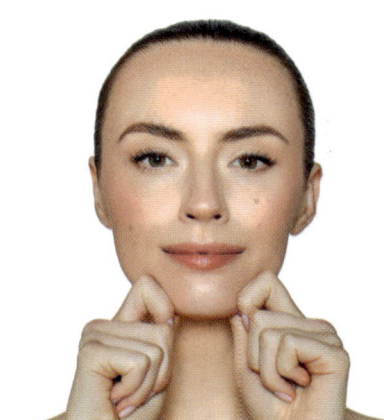

WHEN TO PRACTISE THIS ROUTINE

When your chin and jawline feel soft or undefined, this sequence strengthens deep muscles, boosts lymph flow, and elongates fascia. Step by step, your profile sharpens while your neck feels lighter, lifted, and more open.

4

The Giraffe Kiss
p.128

What it does Lengthens and tones the neck while lifting the lower face.

How Tilt your head back and towards your your shoulder, and pucker your lips into a "kiss" towards the ceiling.

5

The Double Chin Kill
p.128

What it does Strengthens neck and chin muscles for a sharper profile.

How Press your tongue to the roof of the mouth, place a flat hand under your chin, and a fist beneath for resistance. Pulse your tongue up.

6

The Roundabout
p.136

What it does Strengthens the mouth area and smooths nasolabial folds, supporting jawline contour.

How Press your tongue into one corner inside your mouth and circle it around the mouth, pressing into the skin. Reverse direction after 45 seconds.

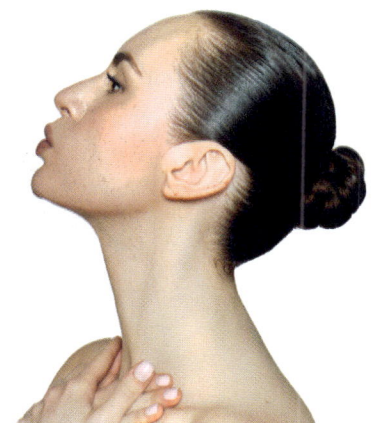
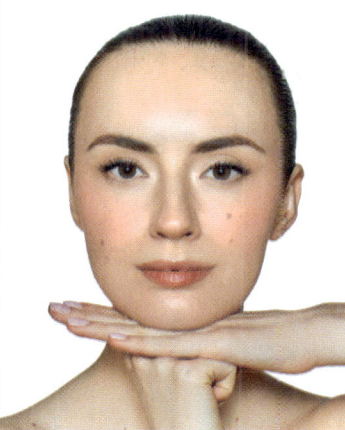
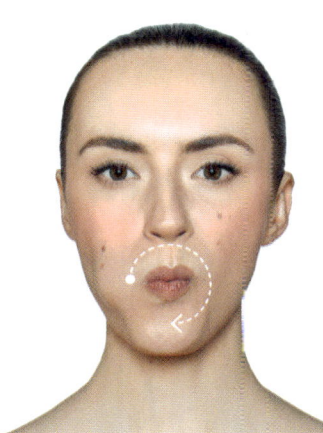

THE ROUTINES

Combat a Sagging Neck

8 MIN

Lift the jawline, activate deeper neck muscles, & restore elegant posture

1

Chest Roll-Ups
p.77

What it does Opens the chest, melts fascia tension, and lifts the tissue that connects directly to the neck and lower face.

How Using thumbs and fingers, gently lift and roll the fascia from the centre of your chest upwards towards the collarbones. Move slowly and steadily across the chest.

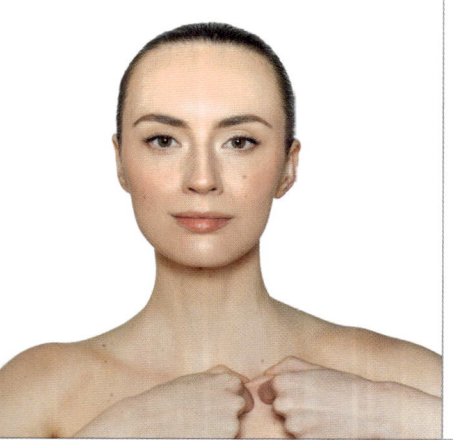

2

The Neck Reset
p.71

What it does Releases tension patterns that cause compression and sagging.

How Interlace your hands behind your back and gently press the back of your head into your hands. Then massage the area where a neck hump might form.

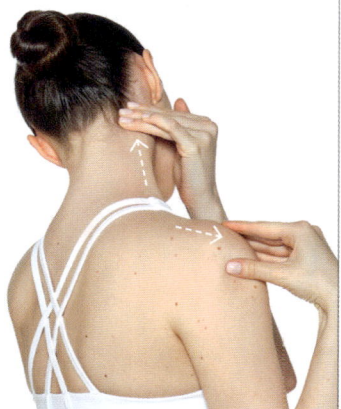

3

The Giraffe Kiss
p.128

What it does Lifts and tones the front of the neck and jawline.

How Tilt your head back and towards your your shoulder, and pucker your lips into a "kiss" towards the ceiling.

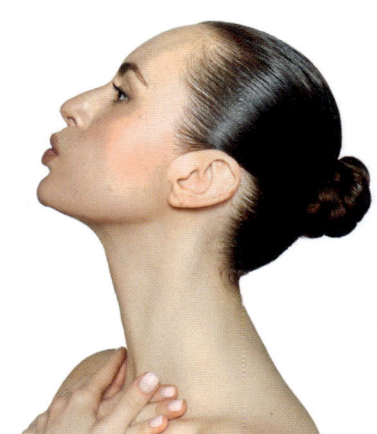

WHEN TO PRACTISE THIS ROUTINE

When posture collapses or hours of sitting create heaviness under the chin, these moves release deep fascia patterns and awaken supportive muscles. With practice, your neck regains length, your jawline sharpens, and your carriage feels elegant.

4

The Double Chin Kill
p.127

What it does Strengthens the tongue-to-neck connection and activates the front line of the neck.

How Press your tongue up into the roof of your mouth while placing one hand flat under your jaw and the other as resistance beneath it. Pulse the tongue upwards for 20 reps.

5

The Jawline Hook
p.115

What it does Releases built-up tension along the jawline and redefines facial boundaries.

How Hook index fingers onto jawline at the chin and press thumbs under the jawbone. Hold for 20 seconds, moving from chin to mid-jaw, then to near the ears.

6

The Mouth Relaxer
p.109

What it does Releases deep tension and tones the neck and jaw, improving jowls, neck wrinkles, and double chin formation.

How Blow out through the mouth with heavy breath, letting lips vibrate in a "Brrrrrrrrr" sound.

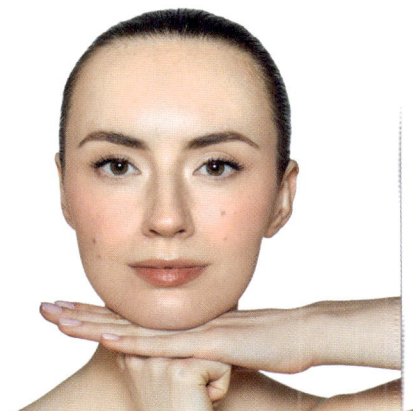
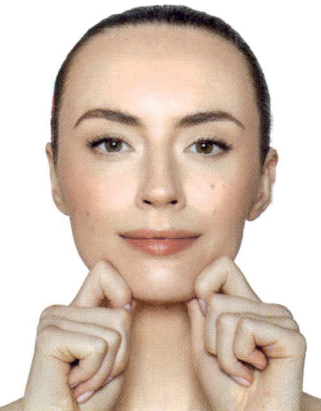
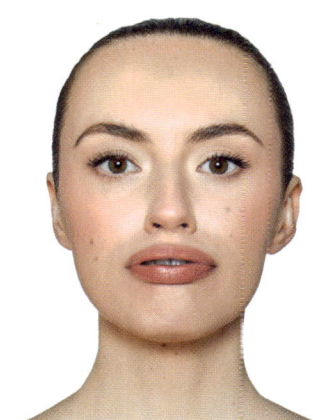

THE ROUTINES

Combat Facial Asymmetry

Balance, align, & harmonize your facial features

7.5 MIN

1

The SCM Release
p.76

What it does Relieves neck muscle tightness that can pull on the jaw and contribute to asymmetry.

How Grasp the SCM between your fingers, tilt your head for a deeper stretch, and massage slowly along its length.

2

The Symmetrical Smile Line
p.134

What it does Improves mouth symmetry and trains balanced smiling.

How Place a clean pen or makeup brush between your teeth, cover with lips, and smile evenly on both sides. Hold, then release and repeat.

3

The Smiling Push Up
p.131

What it does Strengthens the corners of the mouth evenly to support balanced expression.

How Smile as widely as possible with a closed mouth, focusing on lifting both corners equally. Press the smile upwards and hold.

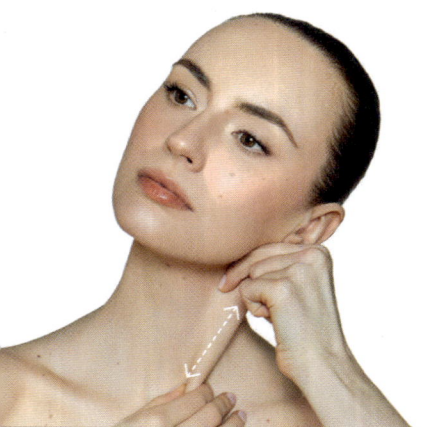
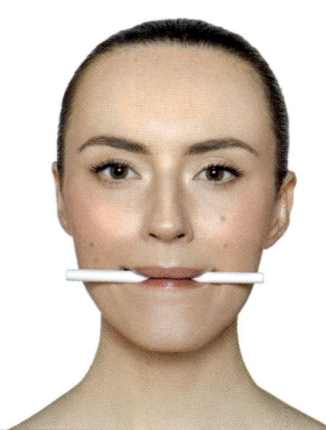
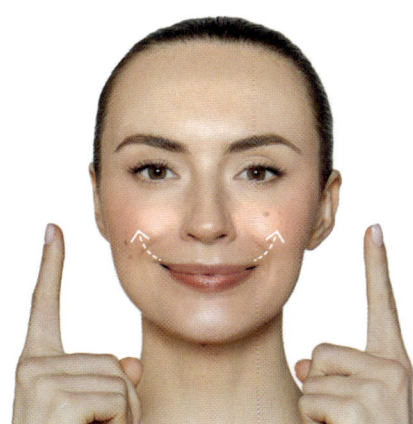

> **WHEN TO PRACTISE THIS ROUTINE**
>
> *When one side of your face feels different to the other, these practices gently guide balance back into muscles and fascia. Over time, small corrections accumulate, aligning features, supporting symmetry, and helping your natural individuality shine through*

4

The Whisper Pose
p.132

What it does Lifts and balances the cheeks and mouth corners.

How Smile widely with mouth slightly open, place index fingers at mouth corners, and gently lift while saying "Sssssss".

5

The Nose Shaper
p.138

What it does Refines nose symmetry by engaging and lifting nasal muscles.

How Lightly press the tip of your index finger under your nose tip. Slowly twitch the tip of your nose up and down.

6

The Eye Symmetry Workout
p.156

What it does Balances uneven eye or brow height through focused activation.

How Hold your stronger eyebrow with your palm to keep it still. Slowly raise and lower the weaker brow, reducing range if forehead wrinkles appear.

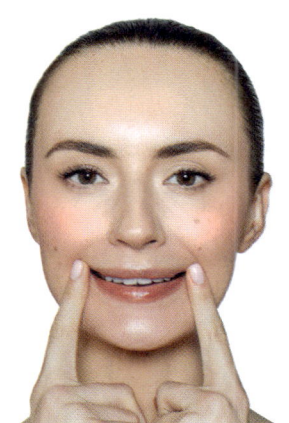
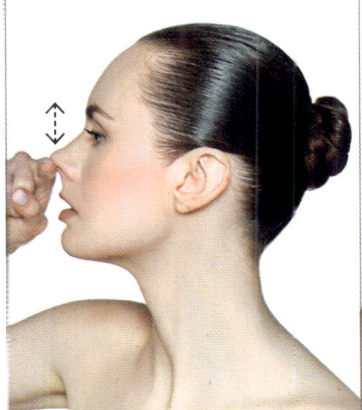
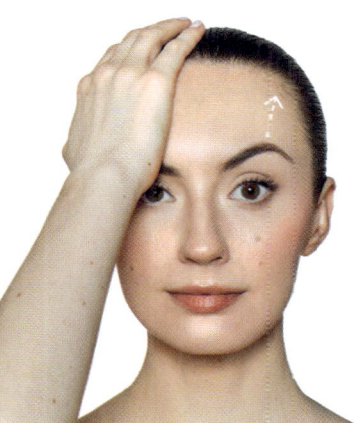

Combat Dull Skin

9.5 MIN

Awaken circulation, brighten your complexion, & bring glow back to your face

1

The Big 6 Lymphatic Activation
p.52

What it does Clears drainage pathways so puffiness can flow out effectively.

How Massage key points in sequence: collarbones, neck, underarms, belly, groin, behind knees.

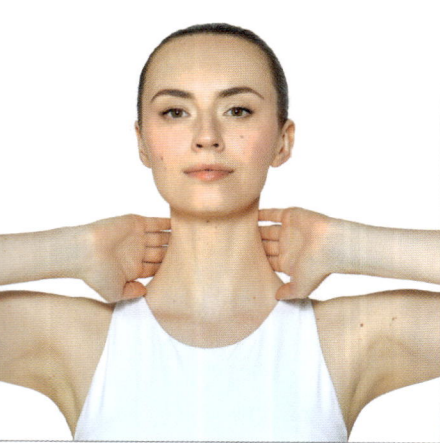

2

The Wow
p.82

What it does Warms up facial muscles, boosts blood flow, and uplifts energy.

How Slowly and exaggeratedly say "Wow," starting with a small "O" shape and expanding as wide as possible without frowning

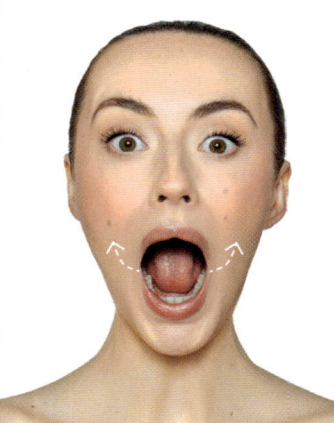

3

The Forehead Tap
p.87

What it does Enhances circulation and softens forehead tension.

How Lightly tap across the forehead, moving from the centre out to the temples.

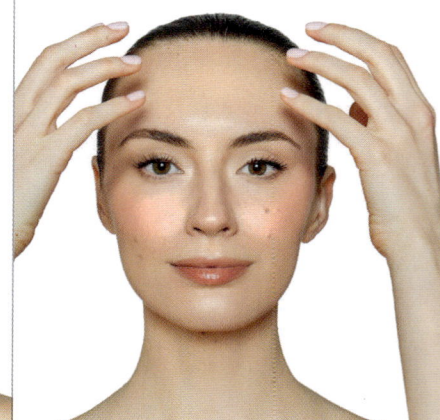

WHEN TO PRACTISE THIS ROUTINE

When your face looks pale, tired, or lacks glow, this quick series reactivates blood flow, awakens fascia, and refreshes skin tone. Gentle tapping and stretching restore vibrancy, leaving your complexion luminous and alive.

4

The Ear Stretch & Wiggle
p.79

What it does Improves circulation, calms the nervous system, and relieves facial tension.

How Gently grasp the outer edge of each ear and stretch lightly upwards, outwards, or back.

5

The Cheek Flick
p.106

What it does Boosts blood flow and revives skin tone in the cheeks.

How Use the pads of your fingers to flick gently but briskly across the cheeks, working from the centre outwards.

6

The Mouth & Jaw Tap
p.114

What it does Activates circulation around the mouth and jawline to restore colour and vitality.

How Tap lightly along the jawline and around the mouth with fingertips or loose knuckles. Keep the rhythm steady and light.

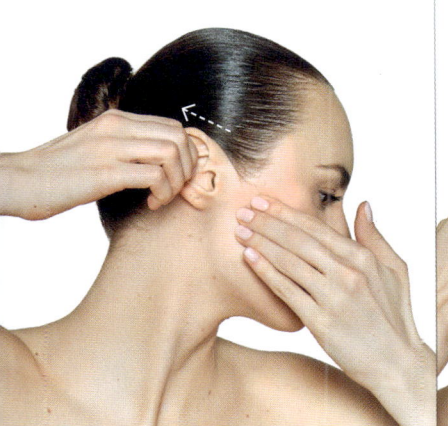
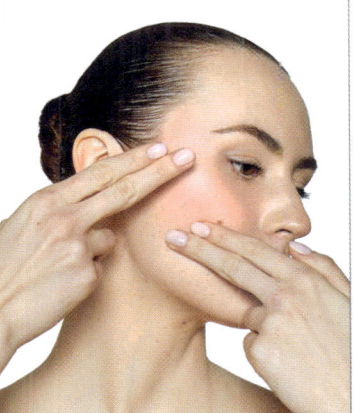
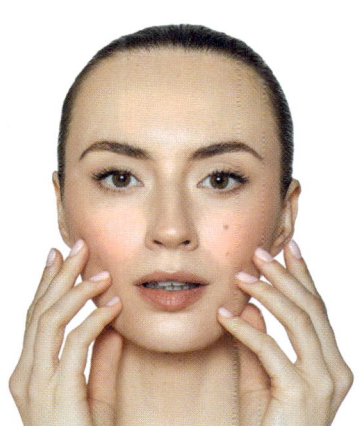

THE ROUTINES

Combat Tension Headache

6.5 MIN

Restore calm to the head, neck, & jaw

1

The Neck Resistance Press
p.73

What it does Strengthens and lengthens neck muscles while releasing tension at the base of the skull.

How Place a band or your hands behind your head. Gently press your head back into the resistance while keeping your neck long and shoulders relaxed.

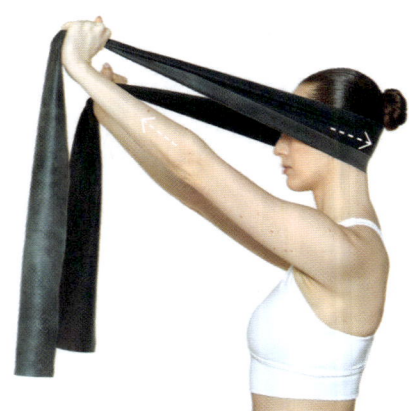

2

The Occipital Bone Massage
p.78

What it does Releases tension where the neck meets the skull – a common trigger point for headaches.

How Use fingertips or knuckles to massage in small, slow circles along the ridge at the base of your skull.

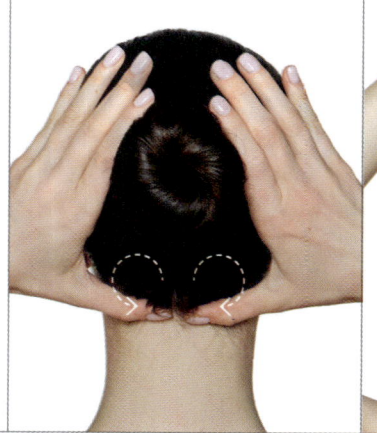

3

The Head Massage
p.81

What it does Stimulates circulation and relieves scalp tightness.

How Using fingertips, massage your entire scalp in small circular motions, applying light to medium pressure.

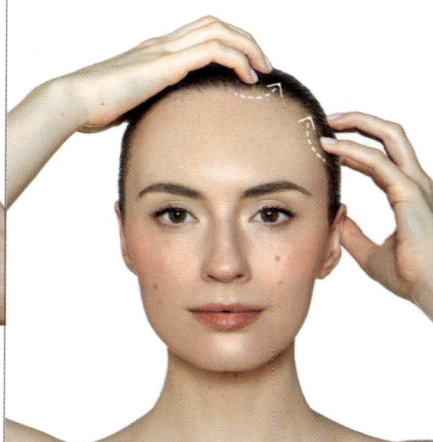

WHEN TO PRACTISE THIS ROUTINE

When stress, clenching, or screen time builds pressure in your head and neck, use this reset. These moves calm tight muscles, release nerve points, and help restore clarity so your face and body can feel balanced again.

4

The Masseter Relaxer
p.83

What it does Releases jaw tension that can radiate into headache pain.

How Glide knuckles slowly from in front of the ear down towards the jawline, with mouth slightly open.

5

The Scalp Shake
p.80

What it does Loosens scalp fascia, improving circulation and calming the nervous system.

How Gently grasp sections of your scalp between your fingertips and lightly shake or wiggle the tissue.

6

The Ear Stretch & Wiggle
p.79

What it does Soothes the nervous system and releases fascia tension connected to the head and jaw.

How Grasp the outer edges of the ears with opposite hands and stretch lightly upwards, outwards or back. Add small wiggles or circles.

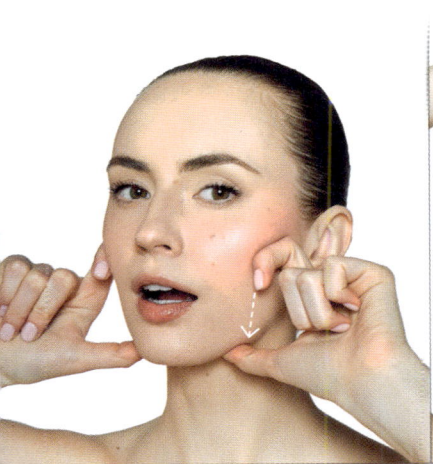
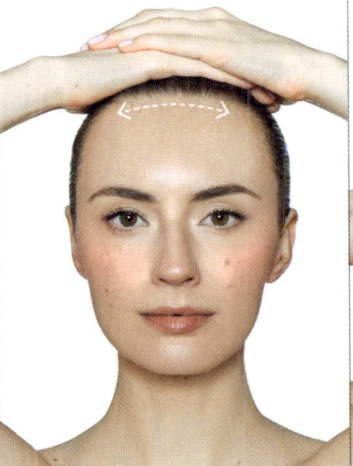
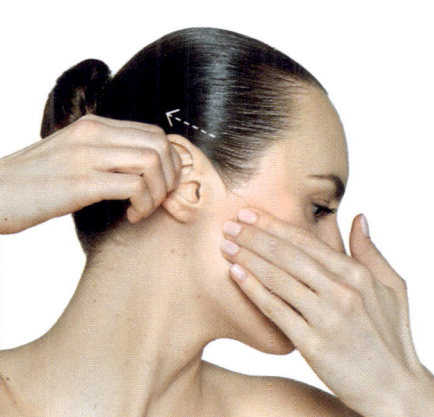

Combat Puffiness

9.5 MIN

Boost lymph flow, flush stagnation, & depuff your entire face

1

The Big 6 Lymphatic Activation
p.52

What it does Clears drainage pathways so puffiness can flow out effectively.

How Massage key points in sequence: collarbones, neck, underarms, belly, groin, behind knees.

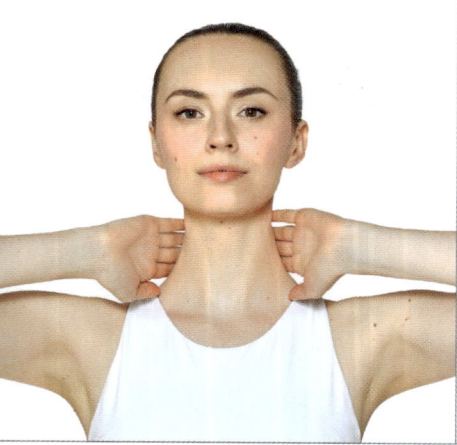

2

100 Jumps
p.54

What it does Stimulates full-body circulation and jumpstarts the lymphatic system.

How Do 100 light bounces or jumping jacks. Keep your body loose, breath flowing, and movements springy.

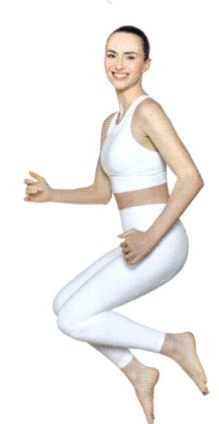

3

The Neck Tap
p.55

What it does Encourages lymph flow from the face down into the body and relieves neck tension.

How Tilt your head, look up, and gently tap from the top of your neck towards your shoulder with the opposite hand. Switch sides after 30 seconds.

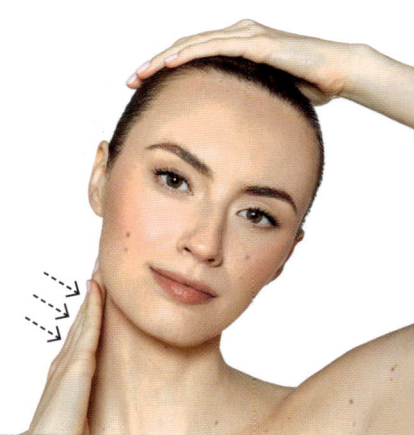

FACE YOGA

WHEN TO PRACTISE THIS ROUTINE

When your whole face feels puffy or stagnant, this routine moves fluid, boosts circulation, and re-energizes the tissues. Simple, intentional movements reconnect body and face, making puffiness fade while glow and definition return.

4

The Wow
p.82

What it does Releases jaw tension that can radiate into headache pain.

How Slowly and exaggeratedly say "Wow," starting with a small "O" shape and expanding as wide as possible without frowning.

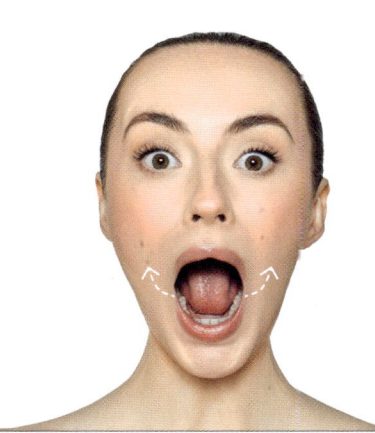

5

The Scalp Shake
p.80

What it does Releases fluid retention and tension at the root (scalp).

How Gently grasp sections of your scalp between your fingertips and lightly shake or wiggle the tissue.

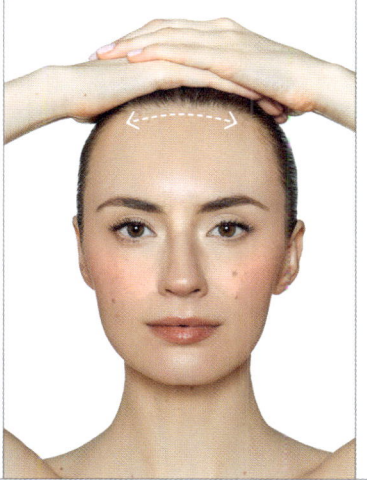

6

The Mini Facelift
p.118

What it does Flushes puffiness, reawakens tone, and brings definition back to the face.

How Use your knuckles or fingertips to glide along the cheekbones, jawline, and temples in slow, sculpting motions. Always work upwards and outwards.

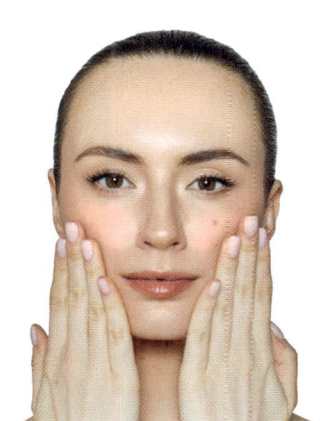

THE ROUTINES

THE

TOOLS

Supporting Tools
Enhancing Your Practice

Your hands are already the most powerful tools you own. Every touch, glide, and movement you've learned so far can be done using nothing but your own fingertips. That's the beauty of face training - it begins with presence, awareness, and technique, not expensive equipment. But sometimes, the right tool can help you go deeper.

This section introduces a selection of optional tools that can enhance your results, support lymphatic drainage, ease fascial tension, and help you reconnect with areas of stagnation or strain. Each one has been carefully chosen for its simplicity, effectiveness, and alignment with the All You Can Face method. From the ancient wisdom of gua sha to the versatility of chilled spoons, these tools invite you to refine your touch, boost circulation, and personalize your routine.

Here's what's important: tools should support your practice, not replace it. No stone, spoon, or suction cup can sculpt your face or "erase" wrinkles overnight. What they *can* do is amplify your efforts, deepen your connection to specific areas, and offer a moment of care that feels grounding and nurturing.

Used with intention, tools can help:
+ Encourage lymph flow and reduce puffiness
+ Release tight fascia and ease muscle tension
+ Boost glow by enhancing microcirculation
+ Activate or calm zones depending on pressure and temperature

You'll find guidance on how each tool works, how to use it properly, and what common myths to avoid. Many people feel overwhelmed by skincare gadgets or get swept up in viral promises. This chapter is here to keep things clear, honest, and rooted in results that come from *consistency*, not gimmicks.

Feel free to explore, but know that nothing in this section is essential. If a tool brings you more joy, ease, or depth in your practice, use it. If not, your hands are more than enough.

Your face responds to care, not trends. And the real magic always comes from within.

COMMON MYTHS ABOUT TOOLS

The following facial tools don't instantly erase wrinkles or dramatically "lift" the face. They also do not reshape bones or melt fat. Their power lies in improving circulation, tension relief, and drainage, supporting your face's natural vitality when used regularly, and creating a subtle, supportive effect over time.

Gua Sha

Stimulate drainage & sculpt your face

Why it exists

Gua sha is a tool rooted in traditional Chinese medicine, designed originally for body treatments to move stagnation and stimulate circulation. When adapted for the face, its purpose is to promote lymphatic drainage, release fascial tension, and enhance microcirculation, supporting a brighter, more sculpted appearance.

Gua sha tools come in various shapes and materials, such as stone (jade, rose quartz), metal, and even resin. While many love stone for tradition, metal tools (such as stainless steel) are hygienic, durable, and less prone to breakage.

How it works

By gliding the tool along specific pathways, you help guide lymph fluid towards drainage points, encourage better nutrient delivery to the skin, and release tight fascia that can pull features out of balance. Done consistently, it can assist with puffiness, dullness, and facial tension.

How to use it properly

+ Clean thoroughly before and after use.

+ Always work on oiled or well-moisturized skin to avoid pulling.

+ Hold the tool nearly flat against your skin (at about a 15–30° angle) for better contact and control.

+ Apply gentle, steady strokes – more pressure does not equal better results.

+ Always move in the direction of lymphatic drainage: outwards towards the ears and down the neck.

+ Avoid broken skin, inflamed acne, or active rosacea areas.

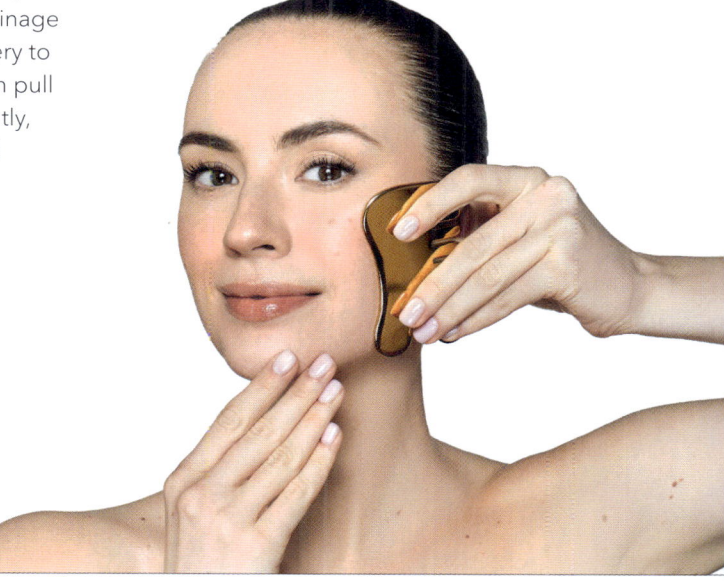

Acupressure Pen

Relax your muscles & release tension

Why it exists
Manual acupressure pens provide a way to stimulate acupressure points without needles, supporting energy flow (Qi), muscle relaxation, and local circulation. This can help release tension that affects facial symmetry and tone.

How it works
The tip of the pen targets specific points on the face and body, applying focused pressure to support muscle balance, nerve activation, and microcirculation. There are electrical versions that emit mild pulses, but the manual, traditional type offers control and simplicity.

How to use it properly

+ Identify key facial points, such as those along the jaw (masseter), between the brows (yin tang), or at the temples (taiyang).

+ Apply gentle, sustained pressure – firm but comfortable.

+ Hold for several seconds, then release.

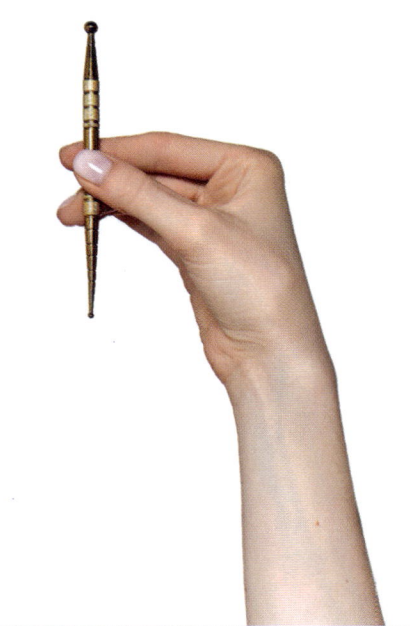

Facial Cups

Encourage healthy circulation & flow

Why they exist
Facial cups are adapted from body cupping, but their purpose is gentler. They're designed to encourage lymphatic drainage, support healthy circulation, and ease fascial restrictions that can contribute to puffiness or a dull complexion.

How they work
The cups create a light suction that lifts the skin and superficial tissue. With constant movement, this promotes circulation and fluid movement without the deep suction marks typical of body cupping.

How to use them properly
+ Use small, soft cups made for the face, not body cups.

+ Apply on well-oiled skin for smooth glide.

+ Keep the cups moving continuously, following lymphatic drainage paths – outwards and upwards on the face, down along the neck.

+ Do not stay in one spot for too long, as this can cause bruising. Strong suction can damage delicate facial vessels.

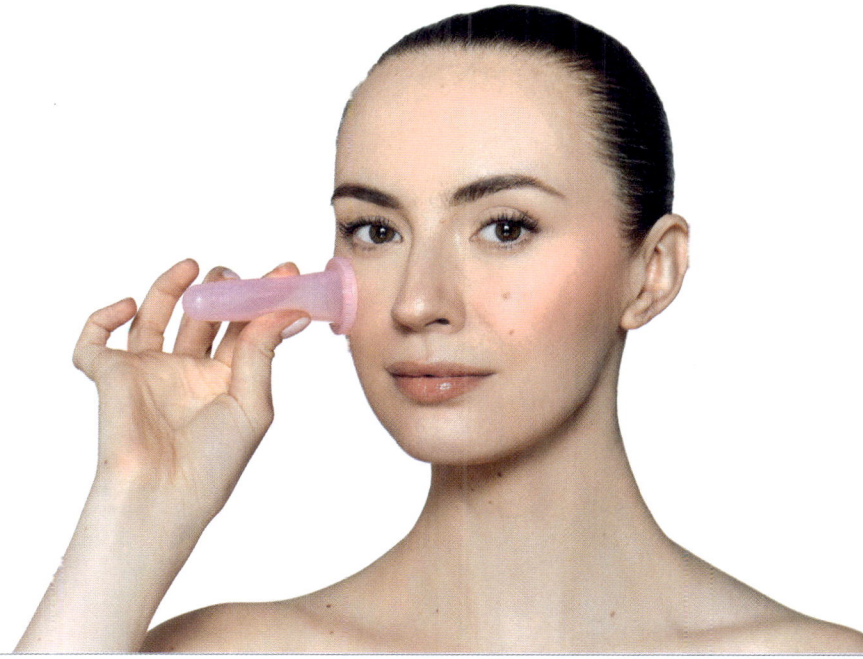

Spoons

Soothe puffiness & smooth out lines

Why they exist
Spoons are an underrated beauty tool that can help with lymphatic drainage, fascia release, and gentle muscle stimulation. Their curved shape fits facial contours, making them great for areas such as under-eyes, the jawline, and cheekbones.

How they work
Used with oil or cream, spoons glide along the skin, helping to reduce puffiness, support circulation, and ease tension. Their temperature - either warmed or gently cooled - can provide additional soothing or depuffing effects.

How to use them properly
+ Use the back of the spoon, never the edge.
+ Apply gentle strokes from the centre of the face outwards, or down the neck for drainage.
+ If using chilled spoons, just like you would a gua sha, ensure they're cool - not icy cold. If warmed, make sure they are comfortably warm - not hot.
+ Clean thoroughly before and after use.

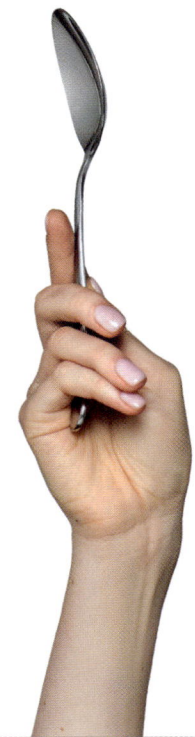

Jade Roller

Calm inflammation & enhance vitality

Why it exists
The jade roller is a traditional Chinese beauty tool that has been used for centuries to support skin vitality, calm inflammation, and promote balance. When used regularly, it helps reduce puffiness, stimulate circulation, and soothe the skin – making it a gentle and accessible addition to any face care ritual.

How it works
The rolling motion supports lymphatic drainage by encouraging fluid movement away from the face and towards key drainage points. It also increases blood flow to the surface, which can brighten the complexion and improve product absorption. The naturally cool stone offers an anti-inflammatory effect, which is especially soothing for tired or puffy skin.

How to use it properly

+ Use on clean, moisturized skin, preferably after applying a facial oil or serum.

+ Start from the centre of the face and roll outwards from cheeks to ears, under-eyes to temples, and brows to hairline.

+ Use the smaller end for delicate areas such as under the eyes or around the nose.

+ Roll down the neck to support full lymphatic drainage.

+ Let the natural weight of the tool do the work – there's no need to press firmly.

+ Clean thoroughly after each use.

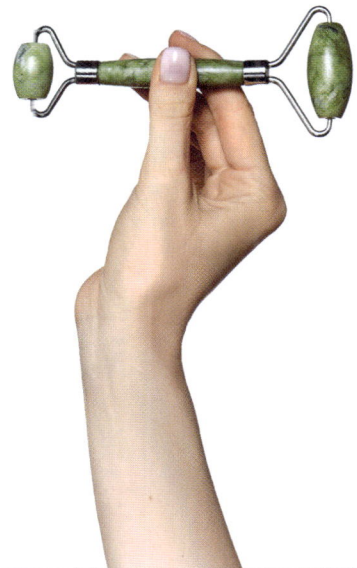

Conclusion

Continuing Your Journey

You have reached the end of this book, but this is only the beginning of your journey. The exercises, tools, and principles you have explored here are not quick fixes. They are invitations to reconnect with yourself, to observe and feel, and to engage with your face and body in a new way.

Your face is not a problem to solve. It is not something to hide or perfect. It is a reflection of your lived experiences, your emotions, your posture, and your inner world. Now, you have the knowledge and tools to work with it – with intention, care, and respect.

What you can do is support your face as it carries you through life. You can bring vitality back through movement. You can ease tension. You can build strength. And through this practice, you can build a kinder, more compassionate relationship with yourself.

Whether you spend ten minutes a day on these exercises or simply bring more awareness to how you hold tension and express emotion, that is progress. Each small act of care adds up. The changes you may see – less puffiness, smoother lines, improved symmetry, a more radiant and confident face – are the natural result of that consistency.

I invite you to take the next step. Join our community @allyoucanface. Share your progress. Inspire others as you inspire yourself. Together, we can change the way we think about beauty – making it about connection, not comparison.

Thank you for allowing me to guide you on this path. I am honoured to share it with you, and I look forward to seeing where it takes you.

With gratitude,
Anastasia

True change doesn't come from chasing perfection, but from recognizing that your individuality is your strength, and that with the right knowledge and simple practices, you can reshape your face and life.

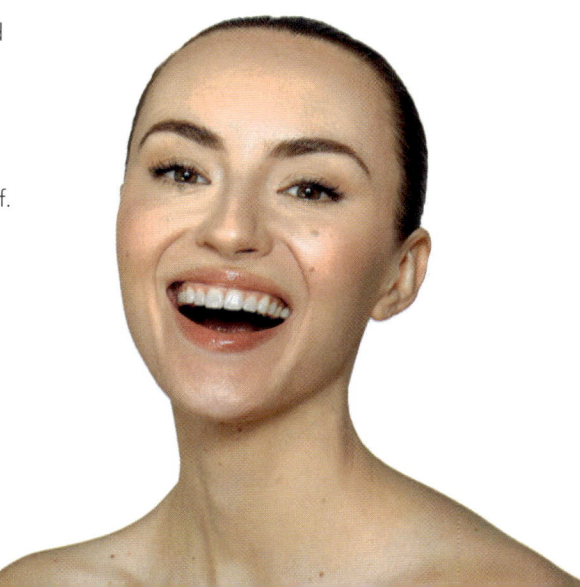

Reccomended Reading

FACIAL ANATOMY AND FUNCTION
3D Anatomy for Manual Therapists, Abby Ellsworth
Facial Action Coding System (FACS), Paul Ekman and Wallace V. Friesen
Atlas of Human Anatomy, Frank H. Netter
Muscles: Testing and Function with Posture and Pain, Florence Peterson Kendall
The Face: Pictorial Atlas of Clinical Anatomy, Radlanski and Wesker
Anatomy of Facial Expression, Uldis Zarins

FASCIA, TRIGGER POINTS, AND BODYWORK
The Concise Book of Trigger Points, Simeon Niel-Asher
Fascial Release for Structural Balance, James Earls and Thomas Myers
The Endless Web, R. Louis Schultz and Rosemary Feitis
Touching Light, Ray McClanahan
Facial Reflexology, Marie-France Muller
Anatomy Trains, Thomas Myers

EMOTIONS, EXPRESSION, AND PSYCHOSOMATICS
Emotions Revealed, Paul Ekman
The Secret Language of the Body, Jennifer Mann and Karden Rabin
The Body Keeps the Score, Bessel van der Kolk
Waking the Tiger, Peter A. Levine
Noverbal Communication: Science and Applications, David Matsumoto
The Polyvagal Theory, Stephen Porges

FACE TRAINING, MASSAGE, AND REJUVENATION
The Book of Lymph, Lisa Levitt Gainsley
Fitness-Training fürs Gesicht, Höfler
The Yoga Facelift, Marie-Veronique Nadeau
Japanese Holistic Face Massage, Rosemary Patten

LONGEVITY, SKIN, AND AGING
Hautnah, Dr Yael Adler
Radical Beauty, Deepak Chopra and Kimberly Snyder
The Positive Ageing Plan, Dr Vicky Dondos
Ancient Secret of the Fountain of Youth, Peter Kelder
Younger Next Year, Chris Crowley and Henry S. Lodge
Lifespan: Why We Age – and Why We Don't Have To, David Sinclair

BEAUTY RITUALS, ENERGY, AND IDENTITY
Move Your DNA, Katy Bowman
Eastern Body, Western Mind, Anodea Judith
The Beauty of Everyday Things, Soetsu Yanagi

Index

A

acupressure pens 198
Advanced Glycation End-products (AGEs) 32
aging 5
  All You Can Face Method
    basic overview 42–47
    posture practice 48–73
    release tension 74–119
    strengthen exercises 120–61
anatomy
  lymphatic system 25
  muscles 18–19
  overview of systems 10–11
  posture imbalances 15
armpits 52, 65, 68
asymmetry
  combat routine 186–87
  conventional treatments 12–13
  fascia and muscle tension 16
  strengthen exercises 132–34, 139, 146, 156, 161

B

belly 53
blood
  circulation 11
  lymphatic stagnation 24
  posture imbalances 14
bones
  anatomy 11
  structural remodelling 30–31
  tongue posture 22
breathing
  mouth breathing 22
  nose slimmer exercise 139
  shallow 24, 33

C

cellular stress 32–33
cervical spine 15
cheeks
  bone remodelling 30
  face map 38
  hollowing conventional treatments 12–13
  muscle atrophy effects 20–21
  sagging conventional treatments 12–13
  sagging routine 172–73
  strengthen exercises 132, 135–37, 141–46
  tension release exercises 85, 102, 104–08
  tongue posture 22
chest
  collapsed, effects 14, 26
  face map 39
  posture practice 61, 64, 67, 69–70
  tension release exercises 77
chewing, asymmetry 16
chin
  double chin conventional treatments 12–13
  double chin routine 182–83
  strengthen exercises 122, 125, 127
  tension release exercises 113
circadian rhythms 32
clavicles 15
collarbones
  face map 39
  lymphatic activation 52
  lymphatic stagnation 24
connection with self 4, 5, 6
cupping 199

D

detoxification 25, 26
diet 33
dull skin
  combat routine 188–89
  conventional treatments 12–13
  lymphatic stagnation 24

E

ear stretch and wiggle 79
emotions
  cellular stress 33
  holding patterns 28–29
environmental pollution 33
expression lines
  conventional treatments 12–13
  muscle atrophy effects 20
eyes
  bone remodelling 30
  drooping eyelids conventional treatments 12–13
  drooping eyelids routine 168–69
  emotional holding patterns 28–29
  face map 37–38
  muscle atrophy effects 21
  puffiness conventional treatments 12–13
  puffiness exercises 94–95, 97, 99, 150, 153
  puffiness routine 166–67
  strengthen exercises 147–57
  tension release exercises 93–101
  tiredness routine 164–65

F

face, general exercises 82, 118–19, 155, 161
face map 34–39
facial cups 199
fascia
  anatomy 11
  lymphatic stagnation 26
  muscle tension 16–17
  posture imbalances 14
fat pads 10, 21
fluid retention 24, 26
forehead
  emotional holding patterns 28–29
  face map 37
  frown line exercises 91–92
  frown lines conventional treatments 12–13
  frown lines routine 170–71
  strengthen exercises 153–60
  tension release exercises 87–93

G

glycation 32
gravity test 39
groin 53
gua sha 197

H

headaches
  combat tension routine 190–91
  occipital bone massage 78
hydration 33

I

inflammation 32

J

jade rollers 201
jaw
  bone remodelling 30
  emotional holding patterns 28–29

face map 39
mouth breathing 22
muscle atrophy effects 20–21
strengthen exercises 123, 125, 142
tension release exercises 83–84, 102, 114–15, 117
tension routine 180–81
jumping 54

K
knees 53

L
laughter liners *see* nasolabial folds
lifestyle influences 32–33
lips
　emotional holding patterns 28–29
　face map 38
　strengthen exercises 128–29, 131, 142, 145
　tension release exercises 110–11
　thinning routine 176–77
lymphatic system
　anatomy 25
　function 11, 26
　posture imbalances 14
　posture practice and activation 50–56, 59–60, 65
　stagnation 24, 26

M
masseter exercises 83–86
mental health 33
mewing 23
mouth *see also* lips; nasolabial folds
　drooping routine 178–79
　emotional holding patterns 28–29
　face map 38
　muscle atrophy effects 21
　strengthen exercises 123, 129–32, 135–36, 142, 146
　tension release exercises 109, 112, 114
mouth breathing 22
muscles
　anatomy 10–11, 18–19

atrophy and support 20–21
bone remodelling 30
fascia and tension 16–17
lymphatic stagnation 26
posture imbalances 14

N
nasolabial folds
　combat routine 174–75
　conventional treatments 12–13
　face map 38
　muscle atrophy effects 21
　strengthen exercises 135–37, 141
　tension release exercises 103
nature exposure 33
neck
　double chin conventional treatments 12–13
　double chin routine 182–83
　face map 39
　head alignment 73
　lymphatic activation 52, 55, 59–60
　lymphatic stagnation 24, 26
　muscle atrophy effects 21
　sagging routine 184–85
　strengthen exercises 122–28
　tension release 71
　tension release exercises 57–60, 63, 116
nerves anatomy 11
nose
　face map 38
　strengthen exercises 138–40
nutrition 30, 33

O
oral posture 22–23
oxidation 32

P
posture
　All You Can Face Method practice 48–73
　bone remodelling 30
　imbalances and facial aging 14–15
puffiness
　combat routine 192–93
　lymphatic stagnation 24
　tension release exercises 83

R
ribs 15, 68
routine building 44–45

S
scalp
　face map 34, 37
　tension release exercises 79–81
screen use 32
shoulders
　lymphatic activation 55
　posture practice 62, 66–67, 69, 71
　rounded, effects 14
skeleton *see* bones
skin anatomy 10
sleep 32–33
smile lines *see* nasolabial folds
social networks 33
spine 15
spoons 200
sternocleidomastoid (SCM) muscle 15, 39, 76
strengthen exercises 120–61
stress, cellular 32–33
sunlight 33

T
tech neck 14, 37
tension
　All You Can Face Method practice 74–119
　face map 39
　jaw routine 180–81
tension headaches, combat routine 190–91
thoracic spine 15
tongue
　mewing 23
　posture 22–23
　strengthen exercises 125–27, 133
tools 196–201
toxins 33
trapezius muscle 15

W
waist 68

References

1. Mehrabian, A. (1972). *Nonverbal Communication*. Chicago: Aldine-Atherton.

2. Adolphs, R. (2002). 'Recognizing emotion from facial expressions: Psychological and neurological mechanisms'. *Behavioral and Cognitive Neuroscience Reviews*, 1(1), 21–62.

   Niedenthal, P.M., et al. (2010). 'Embodied simulation and the human mirror neuron system'. *Behavioral and Brain Sciences*, 33(4), 417–418.

3. World Health Organization. (2023). 'Loneliness and Social Isolation as Public Health Priorities'.

4. Kapandji, I.A. (2008). *The Physiology of the Joints, Volume III: The Trunk and the Vertebral Column*. Churchill Livingstone.

5. Stecco, C., Macchi, V., et al. (2018). 'The anatomical and functional relation between fasciae and muscles'. *Surgical and Radiologic Anatomy*, 30(7), 533–539.

6. Koncz A., Egri D., Yildirim M., Lobko A., Máté E., McVige JW, Schwartz K. 'Postural Responses in Trauma-Experienced Individuals'. *Biomedicines*. 2024 Dec 4;12(12):2766. doi: 10.3390/biomedicines12122766. PMID: 39767673; PMCID: PMC11673034.

Acknowledgements

This book would not exist without the guidance, generosity, and inspiration of so many wonderful people.

To my parents, Lana and Wassil – your unconditional love, sacrifices, and belief in me have shaped everything I do. I'm forever grateful.

To Marcel – All You Can Face wouldn't exist without you. I couldn't ask for a better partner in crime and friend on this adventure.

To my aunt and uncle, Vita and Dima – thank you for having my back during one of the most challenging times of All You Can Face. Your support meant more than words can say.

To my dear friends Isabelle S., Sterre, Brenda, Vilma, Regina, Anja, Lorena, Catriona, Maria, Pauline, Isabelle B., Gaia, Anna, Eve, and Mathilde – thank you for being my first supporters, my cheerleaders, and for believing in me.

To Dejan, for co-creating the name that started it all.

To Reto, for your steady support and wise advice.

To Ugo, for being my mini incubator in the very early stages.

To Nadine, for the beautiful logo that still makes me smile.

To Jascha, for visiting us in Paris and helping us share the magic of face yoga with all of Germany through RTL.

To Madeline, for so generously sharing your transformation with us on TV and inspiring so many.

To Anastasia, for that unforgettable face yoga pyjama party and for inspiring me with your warmth and generosity.

To Anna, for helping me navigate the toughest moments behind the scenes.

To Ruslan, Viktor, and Vitaliy, for being rock-solid in tech – always dependable, always kind.

To Nils, for introducing me to incredible humans and becoming a great friend.

To Dirk, for reminding me to stand tall and defend what matters.

To Nico, for bringing lightness and joy when I needed it most.

To the brilliant team at DK – Zara, thank you for your trust; Chloe, for bringing my ideas to life with such care; Jordan, for your beautiful, thoughtful visuals; and Jasmin, for your kind editorial support. It's been a true joy creating this together.

And to the All You Can Face community – every comment, every photo, every message of transformation has kept me going. You've reminded me that this practice is bigger than me. Thank you for letting me be part of your journey.

About the Author

Anastasia Goron is the founder of All You Can Face, a globally recognized face training method that combines fascia release, facial mobility, and posture rebalancing.

Her mission is to challenge outdated beauty narratives and make facial training as normalized as body training. With over 2 million followers across social platforms and features in Cosmopolitan, RTL, and other international media, Anastasia is leading a global movement that blends education, empowerment, and results.

This book brings her method to life, offering a clear path to transform your face through daily movement, self-awareness, and consistency. Whether you want to soften lines, reduce puffiness, lift sagging areas, or simply feel more at home in your face, All You Can Face gives you the tools to glow naturally, on your own terms.

- www.allyoucanface.com
- @allyoucanface
- @allyoucanface

DISCLAIMER

In this book, I make complex ideas about facial anatomy, posture, and movement easy to understand and apply. I translate knowledge from research and practice into practical techniques you can use in daily life. I am not a doctor, so nothing in this book should be considered medical advice. If you have a medical condition, injury, or are taking medication, please consult your doctor or healthcare provider before trying any of the exercises or practices shared in this book.

PUBLISHER'S ACKNOWLEDGEMENTS

DK would like to thank Karim Kassam, consultant Facial Plastic & Reconstructive Surgeon, for providing valuable insights into facial anatomy, Susan McKeever for proofreading, and Ruth Ellis for indexing.

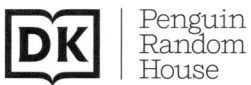

DK LONDON
Editor Jasmin Lennie
Senior Acquisitions Editor Zara Anvari
Senior Designer Jordan Lambley
Production Editor David Almond, Robert Dunn
Production Controller Luca Bazzoli
Art Director Maxine Pedliham
Publishing Director Stephanie Jackson

Editorial Chloe Murphy
Design Hannah Naughton
Illustration Kari Modén
Photography Marcel Nestler

First published in Great Britain in 2026 by
Dorling Kindersley Limited
20 Vauxhall Bridge Road,
London SW1V 2SA

The authorised representative in the EEA is
Dorling Kindersley Verlag GmbH. Arnulfstr. 124,
80636 Munich, Germany

Copyright © 2026 Dorling Kindersley Limited
A Penguin Random House Company
10 9 8 7 6 5 4 3 2 1
001-356869-Jan/2026

All rights reserved.
No part of this publication may be reproduced, stored in or introduced into a retrieval system, or transmitted, in any form, or by any means (electronic, mechanical, photocopying, recording, or otherwise), without the prior written permission of the copyright owner. DK values and supports copyright. Thank you for respecting intellectual property laws by not reproducing, scanning or distributing any part of this publication by any means without permission. By purchasing an authorised edition, you are supporting writers and artists and enabling DK to continue to publish books that inform and inspire readers. No part of this publication may be used or reproduced in any manner for the purpose of training artificial intelligence technologies or systems. In accordance with Article 4(3) of the DSM Directive 2019/790, DK expressly reserves this work from the text and data mining exception.

A CIP catalogue record for this book
is available from the British Library.
ISBN: 978-0-2417-9478-4
Printed and bound in Italy

www.dk.com

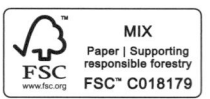

This book was made with Forest Stewardship Council™ certified paper – one small step in DK's commitment to a sustainable future. Learn more at www.dk.com/uk/information/sustainability